MRCP Part 2 Self-Assessment

Medical Masterclass questions and explanatory answers

EDITED BY

John D Firth DM FRCP
Consultant Physician and Nephrologist
Addenbrooke's Hospital
Cambridge

FOREWORD BY

Professor Ian Gilmore MD PRCP
President
Royal College of Physicians

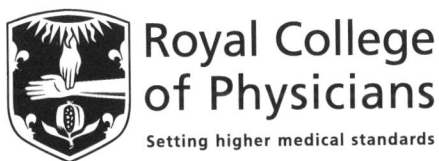

Royal College
of Physicians
Setting higher medical standards

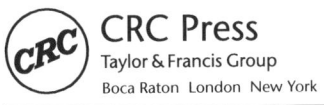

CRC Press
Taylor & Francis Group
Boca Raton London New York

CRC Press is an imprint of the
Taylor & Francis Group, an **informa** business

First published 2008 by Radcliffe Publishing

Published 2016 by CRC Press
Taylor & Francis Group
6000 Broken Sound Parkway NW, Suite 300
Boca Raton, FL 33487-2742

© 2008 Royal College of Physicians of London
CRC Press is an imprint of Taylor & Francis Group, an Informa business

No claim to original U.S. Government works

ISBN-13: 978-1-84619-228-9 (pbk)

The Royal College of Physicians of London have asserted their right under the Copyright, Designs and Patents Act 1998 to be identified as the author of this work.

Visit the Taylor & Francis Web site at
http://www.taylorandfrancis.com

and the CRC Press Web site at
http://www.crcpress.com

British Library Cataloguing in Publication Data

A catalogue record for this book is available from the British Library.

Set by Graphicraft Limited, Hong Kong

Contents

Foreword

Since its initial publication in 2001, *Medical Masterclass* has been regarded as a key learning and teaching resource for physicians around the world. The resource was produced in part to meet the Royal College of Physicians' vision: *'Doctors of the highest quality, serving patients well'*. This vision continues and has led to the compilation of two volumes of self-assessment questions – one of which you now hold in your hands.

The MRCP(UK) is an examination of high international standing and reputation that seeks to advance the learning of, and enhance the training process for, physicians worldwide. On passing the examination physicians are recognised as having attained the required knowledge, skills and manner appropriate for training at a specialist level. However, passing the examination is a challenge. The pass rate at each sitting of the written papers is about 40%. Even the most prominent consultants have had to sit each part of the examination more than once in order to pass. With this challenge in mind, the College and Radcliffe Publishing have produced this compilation of self-assessment questions that were written as part of *Medical Masterclass*, the aim being to help as many doctors as possible in the revision process for the MRCP(UK) examination. I hope you find them to be as beneficial to your studies as thousands of other doctors have; and that you enjoy the challenges they present to your medical knowledge!

Professor Ian Gilmore MD PRCP
President of the Royal College of Physicians
September 2007

Preface

This collection of self-assessment questions and explanatory answers has been drawn from *Medical Masterclass*, which is produced and published by the Education Department of the Royal College of Physicians of London. The questions have been specifically written to help doctors in their first few years of training to test and revise their medical knowledge and skills; and in particular to pass postgraduate examinations, such as the MRCP(UK).

These questions come in the format that is found in both the MRCP(UK) Part 1 or Part 2 examinations. They cover the scientific background to medicine, general clinical skills, acute medicine and the range of medical specialties; all of which candidates will be tested on when they sit their MRCP(UK). The questions collected in this volume will provide a stern test for any such doctor, and how they fare will give them a good indication of where to focus the remainder of their revision if they want to be successful in their upcoming examinations.

I hope that you enjoy using these *Medical Masterclass* self-assessment questions to test your knowledge of medicine, which – whatever is happening politically to primary care, hospitals and medical career structures – remains a wonderful occupation. It is sometimes intellectually and/or emotionally very challenging, and also sometimes extremely rewarding, particularly when reduced to the essential of a doctor trying to provide best care for a patient.

Dr John Firth DM FRCP
Editor-in-Chief
September 2007

List of contributors

Clinical pharmacology

Dr Emma H Baker PhD FRCP
Reader and Consultant in Clinical Pharmacology
Division of Basic Medical Sciences
St George's, University of London
London

Dr Stephen F Haydock MA MB BChir PhD FRCP
Consultant Physician and Director of Acute Medical Services
Addenbrooke's Hospital
Cambridge

Dr Aroon D Hingorani MA PhD FRCP
Senior Lecturer
Centre for Clinical Pharmacology and Therapeutics
University College London
London

Dr D John M Reynolds MA BM BCh DPhil FRCP
Consultant Physician and Clinical Pharmacologist
John Radcliffe Hospital
Oxford

Pain relief and palliative care

Dr G Nicola Rudd MB ChB FRCP
Consultant in Palliative Medicine
Palliative Care Team
Leicester Royal Infirmary
Leicester

Medicine for the elderly

Dr Debra King MB ChB FRCP
Consultant Physician
Department of Medicine for the Elderly
Wirral University Teaching Hospital
Wirral

Dr Claire G Nicholl MBBS BSc DGM FRCP
Consultant Physician and Clinical Director
Department of Medicine for the Elderly
Addenbrooke's Hospital
Cambridge

Dr K Jane Wilson MBBS FRCP
Consultant Physician
Department of Medicine for the Elderly
Addenbrooke's Hospital
Cambridge

Emergency medicine

Dr C Andrew Eynon BSc MBBS FRCP FFAEM
Director of Neurosciences Intensive Care
Wessex Neurological Centre
Southampton General Hospital
Southampton

Professor Paul F Jenkins MA MB BChir FRCP FRCPE
Professor of Acute Medicine
Joondalup Health Campus
Western Australia

Dr Carole M Gavin (nee Libetta) MB ChB MRCP(UK) FRCS(Ed) FCEM MD
Consultant in Emergency Medicine
Salford Royal Hospitals Foundation Trust
Salford

Infectious diseases

Dr Alec Bonington BSc MB ChB FRCP DTMH MD
Clinical Director and
Consultant in Infectious Diseases
Monsall Unit
Department of Infectious Diseases
North Manchester General Hospital
Manchester

Dr Carolyn Hemsley MRCP(UK) MRCPath BM BCh MA PhD
Consultant in Infectious Diseases and Microbiology
St Thomas' Hospital
London

Dr Michael Jacobs MA PhD FRCP DTMH
Senior Lecturer and
Honorary Consultant in Infectious Diseases
University College London Medical School and
Royal Free Hampstead NHS Trust
London

Dr Paul Klenerman MRCP(UK) DPhil
Wellcome Trust Research Fellow
Nuffield Department of Medicine
University of Oxford
Oxford

Dr William Lynn MBBS MD FRCP
Consultant in Infectious Diseases and Medical Director
Ealing Hospital NHS Trust
London

Dermatology

Dr Karen Harman DM MA MB BChir FRCP
Consultant Dermatologist
University Hospitals of Leicester
Leicester

Dr Graham Ogg BM BCh FRCP DPhil
MRC Senior Clinical Fellow and
Honorary Consultant Dermatologist
Oxford Radcliffe NHS Trust
Oxford

Dr Natalie M Stone BA Hons FRCP
Dermatology Consultant
Royal Gwent NHS Trust
Newport, Gwent

Haematology

Dr Kristian M Bowles MB BS PhD MRCP(UK) MRCPath
Consultant Haematologist
Norfolk and Norwich University Hospital NHS Trust
Norwich

Dr David W Galvani MD MEd FRCP FRCPath
Consultant Haematologist
Haematology Department
Arrowe Park Hospital
Wirral

Dr Bronwen E Shaw MB ChB MRCP(UK)
Haematology Consultant
Royal Marsden Hospital
London

Oncology

Dr Mark Bower FRCP FRCPath PhD
Consultant Medical Oncologist
Department of Oncology
Chelsea & Westminster Hospital
London

Dr Graham G Dark MBBS PhD FRCP
Clinical Senior Lecturer
Northern Centre for Cancer Treatment
Newcastle General Hospital
Newcastle-upon-Tyne

Cardiology

Dr Peter E Glennon MB ChB Hons MD FRCP
Consultant Cardiologist
University Hospital
Coventry

Dr Catherine EG Head MA MRCP(UK) PhD
Consultant Cardiologist
Guy's and St Thomas' NHS Foundation Trust
London

Dr Paul R Roberts MB ChB FRCP MD
Consultant Cardiologist
Southampton General Hospital
Southampton

Dr Hamish A Walker BA Hons MBBS MRCP(UK)
Western Infirmary, Glasgow
North Glasgow University Hospitals NHS Trust

Respiratory medicine

Dr Praveen Bhatia MBBS MRCP(Ireland)
Consultant Physician Respiratory and Internal Medicine
Tameside General Hospital
Ashton-under-Lyme

Dr Michael I Polkey MRCP(UK) PhD
Consultant Physician
Royal Brompton Hospital and
National Heart & Lung Institute
London

Dr Veronica LC White BSc MSc MBBS FRCP MD
Vascular Physiologist and Clinical Scientist
Barts and the London NHS Trust
London

Gastroenterology and hepatology

Dr Jane D Collier MB ChB MD FRCP
Consultant Hepatologist
John Radcliffe Hospital
Oxford

Dr John M Hebden MBBS BSc MD FRCP
Consultant Physician and Gastroenterologist
Northern General Hospital
Sheffield

Dr Satish Keshav MB BCh DPhil FRCP
Consultant Gastroenterologist
Department of Gastroenterology
John Radcliffe Hospital
Oxford

Dr Jeremy Shearman DPhil FRCP
Consultant Gastroenterologist
Warwick Hospital
Warwick

Neurology

Dr Gillian L Hall BSc BM BCh MRCP(UK) PhD
Consultant Neurologist
Aberdeen Royal Infirmary
Aberdeen

Dr Aroon D Hingorani MA FRCP PhD
Senior Lecturer
Centre for Clinical Pharmacology and Therapeutics
University College London
London

Dr John P Patten BSc FRCP
Latterly Consultant Neurologist
King Edward VII Hospital
Midhurst
West Sussex

Dr Sivakumar Sathasivam MB BCh MRCP(UK) PhD
Consultant Neurologist
The Walton Centre for Neurology & Neurosurgery
Liverpool

Dr Nick S Ward BSc MBBS MRCP(UK)
Consultant Neurologist
National Hospital for Neurology and Neurosurgery and
Institute of Neurology
University College London
London

Ophthalmology

Dr Peggy Frith MD FRCP FRCOphth
Consultant Ophthalmic Physician
Oxford Eye Hospital and University College Hospital, London

Dr Hamish MA Towler MD FRCPEd FRCSEd FRCOphth
Consultant Ophthalmologist and Lead Clinician
Eye Treatment Centre
Whipps Cross University Hospital
London

Psychiatry

Dr Vincent Kirchner MB ChB FCPsych(SA)
Consultant Psychiatrist
Camden & Islington Mental Health and Social Care NHS Trust
London

Dr Maurice Lipsedge MPhil FRCP FRCPsych FFOM(Hon)
Emeritus Consultant Psychiatrist
The South London and Maudsley NHS Trust
Visiting Senior Lecturer
Department of Psychological Medicine, Guy's, King's and
St Thomas' School of Medicine

Endocrinology

Dr Anna Crown MA MB BChir MRCP(UK) PhD
Consultant Endocrinologist and
Honorary Senior Lecturer
Bristol and Sussex University Hospitals NHS Trust
Royal Sussex County Hospital
East Sussex

Dr Paul D Flynn MA MB BChir MRCP(UK) MRCPI PhD
Consultant Physician in Acute & Metabolic Medicine
Addenbrooke's Hospital
Cambridge

Dr Mark Gurnell BSc Hons MBBS FRCP PhD
University Lecturer and Honorary Consultant Physician
University of Cambridge, Department of Medicine and
Addenbrooke's Hospital
Cambridge

Dr Mohammed Z Qureshi MBBS MRCP(UK)
Consultant Physician
Mid Cheshire Hospitals NHS Trust
Crewe, Cheshire

Nephrology

Dr Nick C Fluck MBBS BSc FRCP DPhil
Consultant Nephrologist and Unit Clinical Director
Medical Renal Unit
Aberdeen Royal Infirmary
Aberdeen

Dr Philip A Kalra MA MB BChir FRCP MD
Consultant Nephrologist and
Honorary Senior Lecturer
Hope Hospital, Salford and
University of Manchester

Professor Patrick H Maxwell FRCP MA MBBS DPhil FMedSci
Chair of Nephrology
Imperial College London
London

Dr Chris A O'Callaghan BA BM BCh MA MRCP(UK) DPhil
Reader and Consultant Nephrologist
Nuffield Department of Medicine and Oxford Kidney Unit
University of Oxford and Churchill Hospital Oxford
Oxford

Rheumatology and clinical immunology

Dr Khalid Binymin MB ChB FRCP MSc
Consultant Physician and Rheumatologist
Southport and Ormskirk NHS Trust
Southport

Dr Hilary J Longhurst MA FRCP PhD FRCPath
Consultant Immunologist and Lead Clinician
Immunopathology and Clinical Immunology
St Bartholomew's Hospital and the London NHS Trust
London

Dr Siraj A Misbah MBBS MSc FRCP FRCPath
Consultant Clinical Immunologist and
Honorary Senior Clinical Lecturer in Immunology
Oxford Radcliffe Hospitals NHS Trust and
University of Oxford
Churchill and John Radcliffe Hospitals
Oxford

Dr Neil Snowden MB BChir FRCP FRCPath
Consultant Rheumatologist and
Clinical Immunologist
North Manchester General Hospital
Manchester

Questions

Clinical pharmacology

Emma H Baker, Stephen F Haydock,
Aroon D Hingorani and
D John M Reynolds *(Editor)*

Clinical Pharmacology

Answers are on pp. 113–115.

Question 1
A 48-year-old woman with a renal transplant is established on ciclosporin, azathioprine and prednisolone to prevent transplant rejection, and enalapril and bendrofluazide for hypertension. After a 14-day course of ketoconazole for oesophageal candidiasis her creatinine is found to have increased from 100 μmol/L to 180 μmol/L. Her deterioration in renal function is most likely attributable to:
A hypertension poorly controlled on enalapril and bendrofluazide
B nephrotoxic effects of ketoconazole
C ciclosporin toxicity due to inhibition of ciclosporin metabolism by ketoconazole
D transplant rejection due to induction of ciclosporin metabolism by ketoconazole
E effect of enalapril on background of stenosis of artery supplying renal transplant

Question 2
Clozapine is an atypical antipsychotic drug that appears to have fewer problems with adverse effects than older antipsychotics. The relative safety of clozapine stems from which one of the following properties:
A low affinity for dopamine D2 receptors
B low affinity for 5HT receptors
C increase in prolactin levels
D does not cause tachycardia
E no effect on white cell counts

Question 3
A 39-year-old woman with a past history of treated hypertension is in her 3rd trimester of pregnancy and requires on-going anti-hypertensive treatment. Which anti-hypertensive would you definitely NOT prescribe?
A hydralazine
B labetalol
C lisinopril
D methyldopa
E nifedipine

Question 4
A 70-year-old woman has severe Parkinson's disease and is on co-careldopa and apomorphine. She complains of nausea and vomiting due to her medication. Which one of the following drugs would you prescribe for these symptoms?
A domperidone
B metoclopramide
C prochlorperazine
D entacapone
E betahistine

Question 5
A 26-year-old woman presents in the 12th week of pregnancy with fever and dysuria. There is no other significant history, but direct questioning reveals a self-limiting rash in the past after taking penicillin. Urine culture reveals a significant growth of Gram negative bacilli. The organism is sensitive to the antibiotics listed below. Which of the following would be the best choice of drug in this situation?
A ciprofloxacin
B gentamicin
C cefaclor
D trimethoprim
E co-amoxiclav

Question 6
You see a woman in late pregnancy who has just been diagnosed with thyrotoxicosis. She is planning to breast-feed her baby after delivery. Which treatment would you recommend for her?
A carbimazole
B blocking dose of carbimazole with added thyroxine
C potassium perchlorate
D propylthiouracil
E Lugol's iodine

Question 7
A 28-year-old man presents following an overdose. Anticholinergic syndrome is suspected. Which one of the following is true of this syndrome?

A tricyclic antidepressants are not a cause
B bradycardia is common
C physostigmine is the treatment of choice
D mydriasis occurs
E urinary incontinence is common

Question 8

A 73-year-old man presents to the Accident and Emergency department with drowsiness and confusion. He is noted to be tachycardic and tachypnoeic. He is not cyanosed, and his pulse oximeter reading is 96% on room air. His wife had been admitted with similar symptoms earlier in the week. Which one of the following is most likely?

A paracetamol overdose
B salicylate overdose
C carbon monoxide poisoning
D cerebrovascular accident
E pneumonia

Question 9

A 79-year-old woman presents to the Accident and Emergency department with confusion, headache and tinnitus. She has recently started on an analgesic for back pain and you are worried she may have taken too much. Which of the following would most likely explain her symptoms?

A paracetamol
B aspirin
C diclofenac sodium
D co-codamol
E codeine phosphate

Question 10

A 35-year-woman presents 6 hours after a deliberate overdose of paracetamol. The paracetamol level is above the treatment line. Thirty minutes after starting an infusion of *N*-acetyl cysteine (NAC) she becomes flushed and hypotensive with a blood pressure of 80/55 mmHg. The infusion is stopped immediately and 500 ml IV 0.9% saline administered over 30 minutes. Which of the following is the correct ongoing management?

A IV chlorphenamine maleate and restart NAC infusion at lowest rate once symptoms resolved
B IV chlorpromazine and restart NAC infusion at lowest rate once symptoms resolved
C IV chlorphenamine maleate and give 2.5 g of oral methionine

D IV chlorpromazine and give 2.5 g of oral methionine
E withhold treatment and recheck paracetamol level at 12 hours

Question 11

A 50-year-old woman has increasing frequency of migraine attacks. You decide to start some prophylactic therapy. Which one of the following drugs would NOT be appropriate for prophylaxis against migraine

A rizatriptan
B sodium valproate
C propranolol
D amitriptyline
E pizotifen

Question 12

A 29-year-old man with a history of epilepsy has been well controlled on carbamazepine and clonazepam for the last 5 years. He now wishes to consider withdrawing from or reducing his medication. Which of the following statements are correct?

A there is about a 60% chance of experiencing a relapse in the first year during withdrawing from anti-epilepsy treatment
B both anti-epileptics can be safely withdrawn simultaneously
C the dose of carbamazepine can be reduced safely by 10% every 2–4 weeks
D he can be advised that he can continue driving during withdrawal from anti-epilepsy treatment as long as she remains free from seizures
E it is likely that he will subsequently require higher doses to regain control with the current therapy, if discontinuation fails

Question 13

You are treating a 72-year-old man with moderate peripheral vascular disease. He exercises regularly but finds that his walking distance is diminishing due to pain. Which drug might help improve pain-free walking distance?

A naftidrofuryl
B cinnarizine
C inositol nicotinate
D simvastatin
E diltiazem

Question 14

A 21-year-old university student complains of difficulty sleeping. She is in the middle of sitting her final exams and would like some medication for a few days to help her sleep. However, she is concerned about potential 'hang-over' effects and would prefer a drug which doesn't cause daytime drowsiness. Which agent would you prescribe?

A diazepam

B midazolam

C promethazine

D loprazolam

E clomethiazole

Question 15

A 74-year-old woman presents with breathlessness. She is a small woman (55 kg) with a chest infection. She is not very unwell, but is in atrial fibrillation at a rate of 170/min. Her electrolytes are normal (K 4.2 mmol/l). As well as treating her pneumonia, you decide to digitalize by prescribing digoxin:

A 0.25 mg orally once daily

B 1.0 mg orally over 24 hours in divided doses

C 1.0 mg intravenously over 20 min

D 0.125 mg orally once daily

E 0.25 mg orally three times daily for one week, then twice daily for one week, then once daily thereafter

Pain relief and palliative care

G Nicola Rudd

Pain Relief and Palliative Care

Answers are on p. 115.

Question 16

A 45-year-old man is dying from non-Hodgkin's lymphoma. He is increasingly agitated and distressed. He is not obviously in pain and has a urinary catheter in situ which is not causing specific distress. He has diamorphine 30 mg in his syringe driver. You are asked to review him. Select the best two options from the list below:

A increasing the diamorphine dose

B adding hyoscine hydrobromide

C no changes to his medication

D reducing the diamorphine dose

E adding midazolam 10 mg to the syringe driver

F giving a stat dose of midazolam

G changing diamorphine to fentanyl

H adding levomepromazine 75 mg to the syringe driver

I giving stat dose of levomepromazine 25 mg

J giving PR diazepam

Question 17

A 56-year-old man with metastatic carcinoma of the prostate has an epidural nerve block for neuropathic leg pain. Following this he is told to stop morphine sulphate continus (MST) but to take some oral morphine sulphate (Oramorph) should he develop any symptoms of opioid withdrawal. Two of these symptoms include:

A sweating

B abdominal pain

C dry mouth

D myalgia

E drowsiness

F cramps

G headache

H myoclonus

I hallucinations

J urinary retention

Question 18

A 40 year old man with complete spinal cord compression at T12 from bone metastases due to lung cancer has not had his bowels open for 6 days. How would you best manage his symptom?

A avoid opioids and other constipating medicines

B prescribe high-dose co-danthramer

C perform rectal examination and prescribe high-dose co-danthramer

D prescribe and titrate polyethylene glycol until bowel movement

E perform PR with enema, prescribe low dose co-danthramer, then administer an enema 3 times per week

Question 19

A 75-year-old woman with metastatic carcinoma of the colon is admitted semi-conscious and dying. Her symptoms had been previously well controlled on oxycodone SR 80 mg bd. What would you do about analgesia?

A nothing at present as she is semi-conscious and not obviously in pain.

B chart prn oxycodone orally

C change to im morphine

D chart prn paracetamol pr

E start a syringe driver with diamorphine

Question 20

A 50-year-old man with metastatic colorectal cancer complains of regurgitation of food and a feeling that it sticks retrosternally. Chest radiograph and upper gastrointestinal endoscopy are normal. Which antiemetic is most likely to be of benefit?

A cyclizine

B haloperidol

C prochlorperazine

D metoclopramide

E ondanestron

Question 21

A frail 58-year-old woman with advanced breast cancer is admitted with abdominal pain and constipation secondary to opioids. Which of the following is the laxative of choice?

A sodium picosulphate

B ispaghula husk (Fybogel)

C senna

D co-danthramer

E lactulose

Medicine for the elderly

Debra King, Claire G Nicholl *(Editor)* **and K Jane Wilson** *(Editor)*

Medicine for the Elderly

Answers are on pp. 115–117.

Question 22
See Figure 1. A 75-year-old woman with a history of long-standing rheumatoid arthritis presents with a 2 month history of malaise, during which time she has lost 6 kg of weight. For the last few months her bowels have become a bit erratic, with occasional constipation for which she has had to take a laxative. Her liver is enlarged about 3 finger breadths below the costal margin and feels firm. Examination is otherwise unremarkable. A CT scan of her abdomen is shown (see Figure 1). The most likely diagnosis is:

A cirrhosis of the liver with ascites

B cirrhosis of the liver

C liver metastases

D liver metastases with ascites

E hepatic amyloidosis

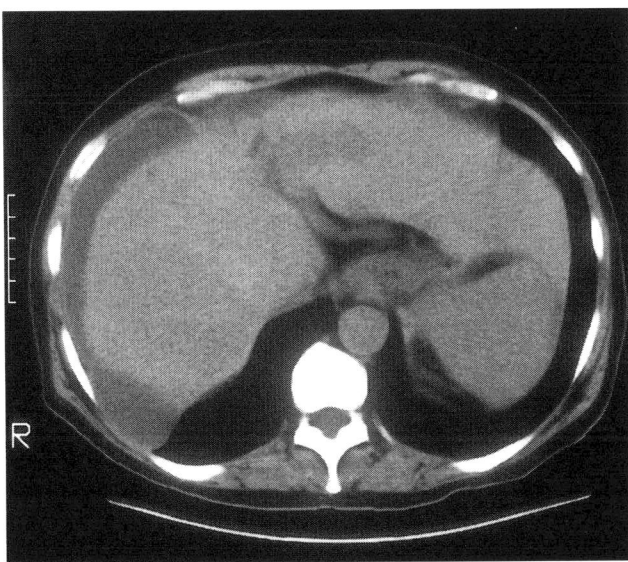

Fig. 1 Question 22.

Question 23
See Figure 2. A 78-year-old woman is referred with complaints of tiredness, decreasing exercise capacity because of breathlessness, and palpitations. A year ago she had a right-sided stroke, from which she made a reasonable recovery such that she was able to return to her home. She lives alone, is socially isolated and has refused offers of support from social services. A picture of her mouth is shown (see Figure 2). The most likely diagnosis is:

A scleroderma

B vitamin B12 deficiency

C hereditary haemorrhagic telangiectasia

D coeliac disease

E iron and folate deficiency

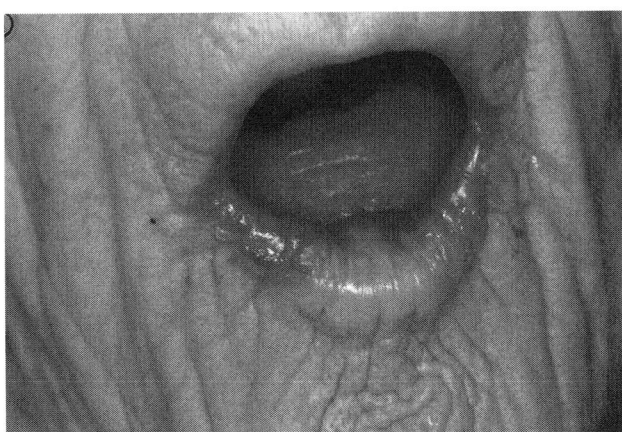

Fig. 2 Question 23.

Question 24
A 74-year-old man has been diagnosed as having idiopathic Parkinson's disease. He is seen in the outpatient clinic and wants to discuss drug treatments available. Which two of the following statements are correct?

A benzhexol has no significant anticholinergic side effects

B benzhexol taken for some time can be stopped abruptly

C benzhexol is especially effective in reducing akinesia

D benzhexol can be safely used in patients with Alzheimer's disease

E amantadine never causes confusion

F levodopa combined with decarboxylase inhibitor crosses the blood–brain barrier

G long term, levodopa may cause dyskinesia and motor fluctuations

H levodopa does not discolour the urine

I apomorphine is a D1 and D2 receptor agonist

J selegiline is a selective inhibitor of monoamine oxidase type A

Question 25

A 74-year-old man is admitted with a history of increasingly poor mobility. Prior to admission he had not been able to get up from his chair. Examination showed bradykinesia, poverty of movement, difficulty in initiating movement and progressive fatiguing and diminishing amplitude of alternating movements. There was no rigidity or tremor, but tone was increased. Which two of the following statements are correct?

A absence of rigidity makes a diagnosis of Parkinson's disease unlikely

B absence of tremor makes a diagnosis of Parkinson's disease unlikely

C the most likely diagnosis is Parkinson's disease

D the cumulative lifetime risk of developing Parkinsonism is 1 in 100

E diagnosis of Parkinson's disease requires extensive laboratory investigation

F diagnosis of Parkinson's disease requires upper body akinesia to be present

G the most likely diagnosis is arteriosclerotic pseudoparkinsonism

H misdiagnosis of Parkinson's disease is uncommon

I cogwheel rigidity does not occur in essential tremor

J rapid progression supports a diagnosis of idiopathic Parkinson's disease

Question 26

A frail 83-year-old man who lives in a nursing home and has type 2 diabetes mellitus is admitted with a chest infection. On general examination you notice that the skin on both heels is pink and boggy. Which statement is true of this situation?

A he is likely to have bilateral deep vein thrombosis

B a minimum 4-hour repositioning schedule should be adopted

C a high carbohydrate diet should be encouraged

D a pressure-relieving support surface should be considered

E there are no validated tools to assess patients at risk of these complications

Question 27

An 87-year-old woman is admitted after being found wandering in her nightie. She says she is looking for her

cat. On examination, she smells strongly of alcohol, but is otherwise well. Her medications include paroxetine for depression, lorazepam for anxiety (she is not sure how many she is taking), cimetidine for longstanding peptic ulcer disease and thyroxine 50 mcg daily. Which medication/ substance can be stopped immediately without problems?

A paroxetine

B lorazepam

C alcohol

D cimetidine

E thyroxine

Question 28

An 87-year-old woman is admitted to hospital after a fall. She has had four falls over the last 6 weeks. Her medications on admission include amitriptyline 75 mg od, temazepam 20 mg nocte, diazepam 2 mg tds, bendrofluazide 2.5 mg od, captopril 25 mg tds, ranitidine 150 mg od and amlodipine 10 mg od. Which one of the following statements is correct?

A tapering and discontinuation of benzodiazepines has not been shown to reduce falls

B tapering and discontinuation of tricyclic antidepressants has not been shown to reduce falls

C reducing the total number of medications to 4 or less reduces the risk of falling

D all older patients with postural hypotension are symptomatic

E falls account for up to 20% of acute hospital admissions

Question 29

A 70-year-old woman with severe Parkinson's disease is on co-careldopa and apomorphine. She complains of nausea and vomiting due to her tablets. Which one of the following drugs should be prescribed for these symptoms?

A domperidone

B metoclopramide

C prochlorperazine

D entacapone

E betahistine

Question 30

A 78-year-old woman is greatly distressed by urge incontinence. Which of the following drugs that might be used to treat her is least likely to cause the side effect of a dry mouth?

A oxybutynin

B tolterodine

C imipramine

D desmopressin acetate (DDAVP)

E flavoxate

Question 31

An 82-year-old woman has recently become incontinent of urine. She is constantly dribbling and feels that her bladder is never empty. What type of incontinence is she most likely to have?

A stress incontinence

B urge incontinence

C overflow incontinence

D functional incontinence

E mixed type incontinence

Question 32

A 74-year-old man is admitted to hospital in a dishevelled state with 'failure to cope at home'. At the ward multi-disciplinary meeting the physiotherapist states that his Barthel Index is 12. Assessment of which of the following does NOT form part of the Barthel Index score?

A feeding

B bathing

C grooming

D reading

E stairs

Question 33

An 87-year-old woman is admitted to hospital with fever and confusion. She does not give a coherent history and at an early stage you decide to perform an Abbreviated Mental Test Score (AMT) to screen for impaired cognition. Which of the following is NOT a question that forms part of the AMT?

A how old are you?

B what is the time?

C what year is it?

D what were the years of the First World War?

E name of the present prime minister?

Question 34

A 70-year-old man is referred for increasing forgetfulness. On closer questioning, he admits to some urinary incontinence and unsteadiness on walking. He smokes 40 cigarettes a day and has been a heavy drinker in the past. What is most likely diagnosis?

A alcoholic cerebellar degeneration

B Alzheimer's disease

C frontotemporal dementia

D multi-infarct dementia

E normal pressure hydrocephalus

Question 35

An 84-year-old man presents with a 6-month history of increasing confusion, visual hallucinations, reduced mobility and falls. Which type of dementia fits this history best?

A Alzheimer's disease

B Pick's disease

C dementia with Lewy bodies

D Parkinson's disease

E vascular dementia

Question 36

An 82-year-old man is admitted following a fall. The physiotherapist thinks he looks Parkinsonian and asks for your opinion. Which of the following is most supportive of a diagnosis of Parkinson's disease?

A his tremor is most disabling when he is drinking his tea

B his neck is extended and he has a surprised expression, despite paucity of facial movement

C the tremor is worse in his left arm and leg

D you elicit a positive glabellar tap

E you notice marked oro-facial dyskinesia

Emergency medicine

C Andrew Eynon, Paul F Jenkins *(Editor)* and Carole M Gavin

Emergency Medicine

Answers are on pp. 117–121.

Question 37

A 48-year-old man with no significant past medical history and on no regular medication presents with central chest pain that radiates to his neck. For 48 hrs prior to admission he has felt feverish, with headache and generalized aches in his muscles and joints. He has smoked 20 cigarettes a day for about 30 years. His father died at the age of 74 years following a heart attack. He does not look unwell, but is febrile (37.8 degrees). Examination is otherwise unremarkable. His ECG is shown (see Figure 3). The most likely diagnosis is:

A acute inferior myocardial infarction

B acute inferior myocardial infarction with lateral extension

C pericarditis

D pulmonary embolism

E myocarditis

Question 38

A 68-year-old man presents with one hour of central chest pain. His ECG is shown (see Figure 4). The diagnosis is:

A pericarditis

B acute inferior myocardial infarction with posterior extension

C acute anterior myocardial infarction with lateral extension

D acute anterior myocardial infarction

E acute inferior myocardial infarction

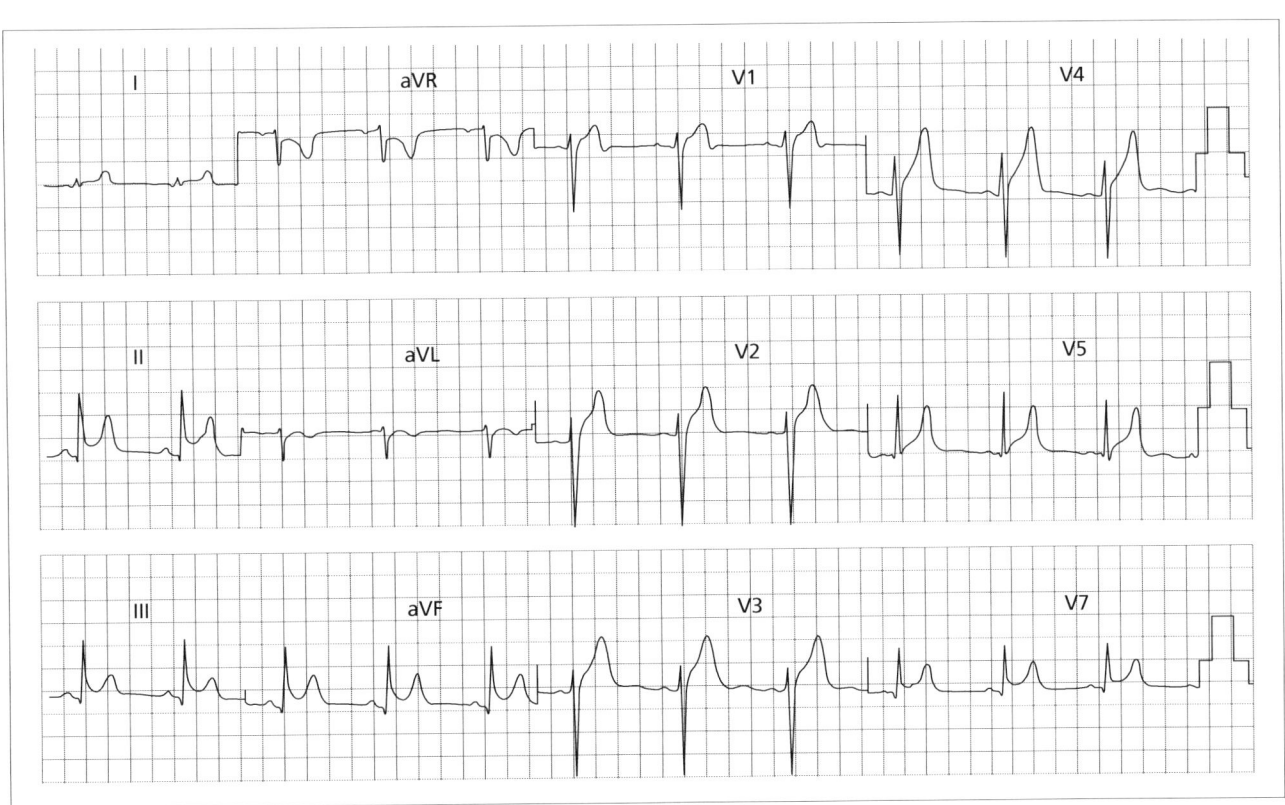

Fig. 3 Question 37.

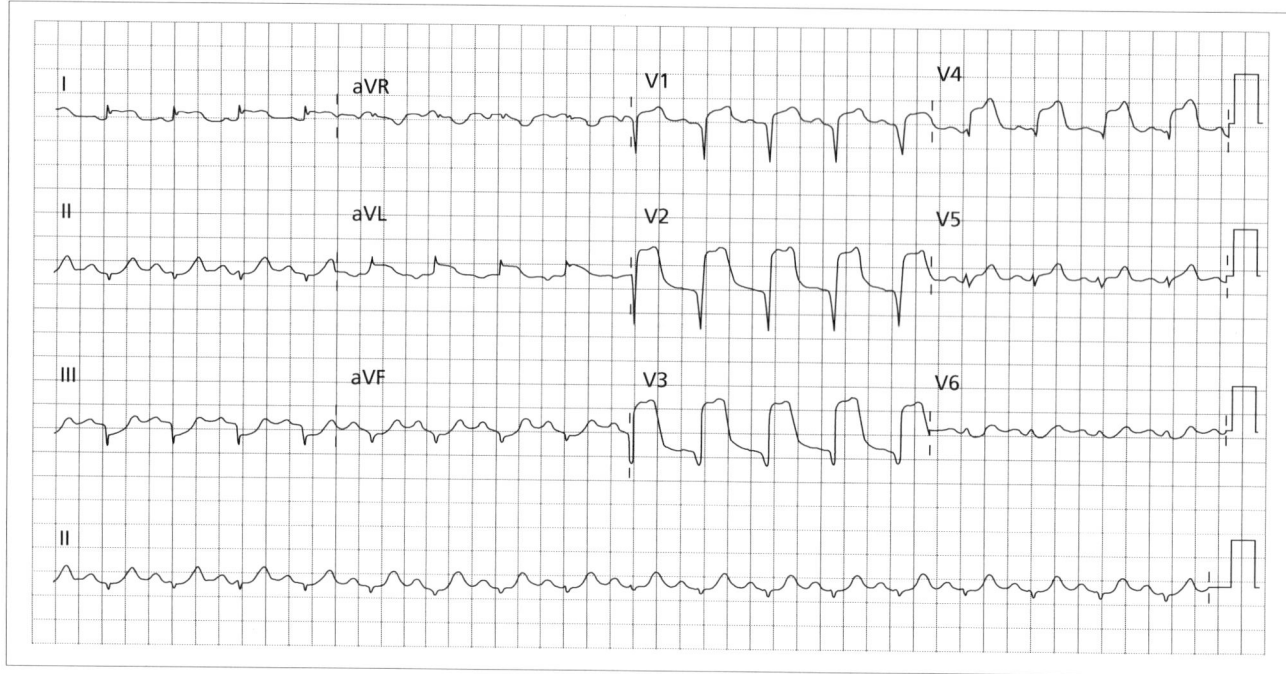

Fig. 4 Question 38.

Question 39

A 48-year-old man presents with 40 minutes of cardiac chest pain. Which two of the following ECG criteria are indications for thrombolysis?

A 2 mm or more elevation of the ST segment in any one standard ECG lead

B atrial fibrillation

C 2 mm or more ST segment depression in two or more standard ECG leads

D 2 mm or more elevation of ST segments in two or more contiguous praecordial leads

E new right bundle branch block

F ventricular tachycardia

G 1 mm or more elevation of ST segments in two or more standard ECG leads

H 2 mm or more elevation of ST segments in any two ECG leads

I 1 mm or more elevation of ST segments in any two ECG leads

J 1 mm or more elevation of ST segments in two or more contiguous praecordial leads

Question 40

A 22-year-old man presents to the Accident and Emergency department claiming to have taken a large quantity of paracetamol 24 hours previously. He washed the tablets down with vodka. Which two of the following statements are correct?

A measuring paracetamol levels at 24 hours is of no use

B N-acetyl cysteine should be witheld until plasma paracetamol levels are known.

C the prognostic accuracy of the treatment nomogram is less certain at 24 hours post-ingestion.

D methionine can be given if the patient is intolerant of N-acetyl cysteine (NAC).

E clinical symptoms may occur > 24 hours post-ingestion.

F if the urea and electrolytes are normal, the patient can be sent home.

G even at 24 hours, activated charcoal should be given as gastric transit time is prolonged by paracetamol.

H the measurement of alanine transferase is of prognostic value.

I if he drank more than two units of alcohol with the overdose, he is at greater risk.

J if he is obese, he is at greater risk from the effects of the overdose

Question 41

A 40-year-woman presents after a deliberate overdose of paracetamol. Which two of the following are suggestive of the development of acute liver failure 48 hours after a paracetamol overdose?

A prothrombin time > 60 seconds, control 12 seconds
B albumin > 30 g/ litre
C alanine aminotransferase (ALT) ten times upper limit of laboratory normal range
D evidence of metabolic acidosis
E hyperglycaemia
F hypokalaemia
G elevated C-reactive protein (CRP)
H leucocytosis
I erythrocyte sedimentation rate (ESR) > 50 mm/hr
J thrombocytosis

Question 42

A 22-year-old woman with known severe asthma presents to the emergency department complaining of acute breathlessness for the last 4 hours. She has had no response from her ordinary medication and is getting distressed. The ambulance crew have given 100% oxygen and a salbutamol nebuliser. Which two of the following statements concerning the management of acute severe asthma are correct?
A aminophylline improves the ventilation/perfusion mismatch
B hyperkalaemia commonly follows treatment with beta-2 agonists
C patients require high right ventricular filling pressures
D 28–35% oxygen should be used for patients with hypercapnia to avoid progressive hypoventilation
E intravenous beta-2 agonists are contraindicated as they exacerbate tachycardia
F the most important investigation is the peak expiratory flow rate
G a normal arterial carbon dioxide concentration suggests the alternative diagnosis of hysterical hyperventilation
H low dose diazepam is useful for alleviating anxiety
I the degree of pulsus paradoxus correlates with the severity of the attack
J absence of wheeze excludes the diagnosis

Question 43

A 72-year-old woman has been admitted to the ward via the Emergency Department. She was found collapsed at home, semiconscious. Her Glasgow coma score (GCS) is currently 10 and she is receiving oxygen via a venturi mask. You notice that she has stridor with marked inspiratory effort. Which two of the following statements regarding basic airway management are correct?
A the length of an oropharyngeal airway should correspond to the length of the patient's little finger

B oropharyngeal airways are contraindicated in patients with a base of skull fracture
C patients with preserved laryngeal reflexes will not tolerate a nasopharyngeal tube
D insertion of an oropharyngeal airway can trigger laryngospasm
E a nasopharyngeal airway cannot be used if the nose is fractured
F both nasopharyngeal and oropharyngeal airways can provide a definitive airway for comatose patients
G nasopharyngeal and oropharyngeal airways should be used when a jaw thrust is contraindicated
H the diameter of a nasopharyngeal tube should be similar to the diameter of the patient's little finger
I a head tilt chin lift produces less neck movement than a jaw thrust manoeuvre
J vomitus should be removed from the airway using a blind finger-sweep

Question 44

Non-invasive methods of ventilation (NIV) are increasingly used for patients with a variety of acute and chronic medical conditions. A 75-year-old smoker with end-stage chronic obstructive pulmonary disease is admitted. He has been using NIV at home. Which two of the following statements regarding non-invasive ventilation are correct?
A It is not indicated for patients with terminal conditions
B It should only be used with a nasogastric tube in situ
C It reduces expiratory effort
D It can cause facial skin necrosis
E It can be used for comatose patients
F It may be of benefit for patients with sleep apnoea
G It increases the work of breathing
H It should only be used if the patient has a definitive airway
I It can be used only for type 1 respiratory failure
J It reduces functional residual capacity

Question 45

A 67-year-old man is on coronary care following an inferior myocardial infarct. He has had a temporary transvenous pacemaker inserted for Mobitz type II heart block. He suddenly becomes light-headed with chest pain. The cardiac monitor shows complete heart block with a rate of 20 bpm. What should be your first two actions?
A call the cardiac arrest team
B ask him to cough repeatedly

C give a precordial thump

D check the lead connections on the pacemaker

E institute external pacing

F obtain a 12 lead electrocardiogram

G increase the pacemaker voltage to maximum

H start an isoprenaline infusion

I give streptokinase 1.5 MU intravenously

J give morphine 5–10 mg intravenously

Question 46

A 40-year-old woman presents four hours after an overdose of amitriptyline and diazepam. On examination her Glasgow Coma Scale score is 10. She has dilated pupils, a blood pressure of 100/70 mmHg and a pulse of 140 beats per minute. Her SaO_2 (pulse oximetry) is 95% and her blood glucose (finger prick test) is 7.0 mmol/l. Which is the most appropriate other immediate investigation?

A CT brain scan

B serum urea and electrolytes

C ECG

D serum paracetamol level

E serum salicylate level

Question 47

A 35-year-old woman presents 2 hours after collapsing at home with severe headache. On examination she is drowsy and has neck stiffness. Her temperature is 37.5°C. She has a mild right hemiparesis. Which of the following is the most appropriate first diagnostic investigation?

A CT brain scan

B lumbar puncture and examination of the cerebrospinal fluid

C four-vessel angiography

D MR angiogram

E MR brain scan

Question 48

A 50-year-old man presents with lethargy and palpitations. His ECG shows tented T waves, small/absent P waves, and broad QRS complexes. Investigations reveal:

Serum sodium	144 mmol/L (Normal range: 137–144)
Serum potassium	7.9 mmol/L (3.5–4.9)
Serum bicarbonate	9 mmol/L (20–28)
Serum urea	40.5 mmol/L (2.5–7.5)
Serum creatinine	510 µmol/L (60–110)

The best immediate therapy is:

A intravenous calcium gluconate

B intravenous dextrose and insulin

C intravenous sodium bicarbonate

D nebulised salbutamol

E rectal calcium resonium

Question 49

A 75-year-old man is admitted to hospital. He is receiving warfarin as prophylaxis following a DVT. His international normalised ratio (INR) has been stable at 2–2.5 for the past 8 weeks. While in hospital his INR increases to >8: which of the following drugs prescribed in hospital could cause his increased INR?

A ciprofloxacin

B aspirin

C carbamazepine

D rifampicin

E co-dydramol

Question 50

A 50-year-old woman presents to the emergency department with a short history of severe occipital headache, vomiting and impaired balance. Her past medical history includes hypertension. On examination she has nystagmus to the right, ataxia of her right limbs and gait ataxia. What is the most likely diagnosis?

A basal ganglia haemorrhage

B subdural haemorrhage

C left temporal lobe haemorrhage

D pontine haemorrhage

E cerebellar haemorrhage

Question 51

A 48-year-old man is admitted to hospital with an anterior myocardial infarct. He receives treatment with thrombolysis, aspirin, a beta blocker and a statin. He makes good progress and is about to be discharged on day 7 when he develops chest pain. This is different in nature from the pain that precipitated his admission. You cannot decide clinically whether it is ischaemic cardiac pain. In deciding how to investigate, which one of the following statements regarding troponins is correct?

A elevated plasma concentrations are specific markers for ischaemic heart disease

B elevated plasma concentrations would typically be found two weeks after an acute myocardial infarction

C the sensitivity of troponins for cardiac muscle damage is similar to that of CK-MB

D reduced plasma concentrations are typically found in patients who are in atrial fibrillation

E troponins have a key role in the decision regarding thrombolysis in patients presenting with chest pain

Question 52

A 33-year-old woman presents with sudden onset pleuritic chest pain that came on while she was lifting her 18-month-old son. She complains of feeling short of breath. She is otherwise fit and well, is on no medication, but smokes 10 cigarettes per day. Clinical examination is normal, as are chest x-ray and resting ECG. Pulse oximetry reveals that her oxygen saturation breathing room air is 97%. A Vidas D-dimer is less than 500 ng/ml, i.e. within the normal range. The most likely diagnosis is:

A musculoskeletal chest pain

B pericarditis

C pulmonary embolism

D atypical pneumonia

E unstable angina

Question 53

A 55-year-old man with a history of severe asthma and ischaemic heart disease is brought to the Emergency Department complaining of palpitations and syncope. On examination he has a weak, regular pulse with a rate of 180 / minute with a blood pressure of 110/70 mmHg. A 12 lead ECG reveals a broad complex tachycardia. Which of the following statements is correct?

A absence of capture or fusion beats on a long rhythm strip is strongly suggestive of supraventricular tachycardia (SVT) with aberrant conduction

B SVT is more likely than ventricular tachycardia (VT) if the patient gives a history of recent myocardial infarction

C intravenous adenosine should be used to distinguish SVT from VT

D QRS calibre greater than 0.2s is usually indicative of VT

E SVT with aberrant conduction is unlikely if a recent ECG showed no evidence of bundle branch block

Question 54

A 45-year-old man with chronic alcoholic liver disease was admitted earlier in the day following a large haemate-

mesis. He was treated with intravenous terlipressin and urgent endoscopy was arranged after initial fluid resuscitation and correction of a mild coagulopathy with fresh frozen plasma. Endoscopy revealed bleeding oesophageal varices, which were injected with sclerosant with apparently good effect. He has been stable on the ward for the past 6 hours, but you are called to see him in the early hours of the following morning because he has had a further 500 ml haematemesis, and his blood pressure has dropped from 130/90 mmHg to 90/50 mmHg. Which of the following measures would be most appropriate in addition to fluid resuscitation?

A urgent repeat endoscopy and sclerotherapy

B change terlipressin to octreotide

C administer 10 mg vitamin K intravenously

D insert Sengstaken tube, inflate gastric balloon and apply traction

E urgent surgical intervention

Question 55

A 45-year-old man with a history of alcohol-related chronic liver disease presents following a 400 ml fresh haematemesis. On examination he is jaundiced with palmar erythema and marked ascites. Pulse is 120 beats per minute and blood pressure 100/70 mmHg. In addition to fluid resuscitation, which of the following treatments is most likely to be beneficial in his initial management, while awaiting upper GI endoscopy?

A ranitidine 50 mg intravenously

B omeprazole 40 mg intravenous bolus

C tranexamic acid 1 g intravenously

D terlipressin 2 mg intravenous bolus

E propranolol 40 mg orally

Question 56

A 26-year-old woman presents with a week's history of progressive numbness and weakness in her lower limbs. Which of the following suggests a diagnosis of Guillain-Barré syndrome (GBS)?

A optic atrophy on fundoscopy

B a sensory level

C ankle weakness with saddle area sensory loss

D autonomic dysfunction

E proximal weakness > distal

Question 57

A frail 73-year-old woman is admitted via the Accident and Emergency department with agitation, restlessness and confusion. On examination she is apyrexial and has no chest signs. Abdominal examination is normal and rectal examination reveals a small amount of normal stool. Her son reports that she had been staying with him for a long weekend just to give her a break, but unfortunately she had forgotten to bring her medications with her. He says that she has a long history of agitation and anxiety. Her blood tests are all normal. Urine dipstick testing for nitrites and leucocytes is negative. The most likely cause for her confused state is:

A urinary tract infection
B chest infection
C alcohol withdrawal
D constipation
E benzodiazepine withdrawal

Question 58

A 47-year-old woman with a past history of relapsing-remitting multiple sclerosis presents to the acute medical take following a flare-up of her condition. Which of the following statements regarding steroid treatment is NOT true?

A corticosteroid treatment may limit the duration of visual loss due to optic neuritis
B avascular necrosis of the femoral head is a recognised complication of corticosteroid treatment
C corticosteroid treatment may reduce the frequency of future relapses
D oral corticosteroid treatment has no impact on rate of recovery from a relapse
E 1 g methylprednisolone daily for 3 days is an appropriate dose

Question 59

A 28-year-old woman with type I diabetes mellitus develops abdominal pain and vomiting after eating a stale chicken sandwich. She presents to hospital two days later. Which of the following statements concerning diabetic ketoacidosis is NOT correct?

A it may present as an acute abdomen
B serum amylase may be elevated without evidence of pancreatitis
C the white cell count may be elevated without evidence of infection
D the anion gap is normal
E although serum potassium is often raised, total body potassium is reduced

Question 60

An 18-year-old woman is brought to the Accident and Emergency department by a friend, who says that she has been ill for 24 hours with 'flu-like symptoms and headache. She is unwell, drowsy and has a purpuric rash on her arms. Your immediate action is to:

A order a CT scan of her brain
B perform a lumbar puncture
C take blood cultures and await result
D give aciclovir 10 mg/kg intravenously
E give cefotaxime 2 g intravenously

Question 61

A man is brought to the Accident and Emergency department by ambulance. He is unconscious (GCS 5) with pin-point pupils and a slow respiratory rate. Immediate specific treatment should be:

A naloxone (0.4 mg) intravenously, repeated if no effect
B N-acetyl cysteine (150 mg/kg over 15 min) intravenously, then 50 mg/kg over 4 hours, then 100 mg/kg over 16 hours
C dextrose (50 ml of 50% solution) intravenously, repeated if no effect
D naloxone (4 mg) intravenously, repeated if no effect
E insert stomach tube (after securing airway) and give activated charcoal

Question 62

A 38-year-old man presents with acute renal failure and serum creatinine 988 µmol/l. A house physician performs arterial blood gas analysis (breathing air) and finds pH 7.12, pO_2 12.8 kPa, pCO_2 3.2 kPa, BE –12 mmol/l. He asks you what a base excess of –12 means. You reply:

A it means that the serum bicarbonate concentration is 12 mmol/l
B it means that the serum bicarbonate concentration is 12 mmol/l below normal
C it means that the pH is 0.12 units below the lower limit of the normal range for the machine being used
D an algorithm is used to predict what pH would arise in normal blood in the presence of the pCO_2 actually measured, the base excess being the amount of acid that would have to be added or removed to obtain the pH actually measured
E an algorithm is used to predict what pH would arise in normal blood in the presence of the pCO_2 actually measured, the base excess being the amount of base that

would have to be added or removed to obtain the pH actually measured

Question 63

A 38-year-old asthmatic woman presents with an acute attack. Her arterial blood gases breathing air are as follows: pH 7.36, pO_2 9.8 kPa, pCO_2 5.2 kPa. These are most likely to mean:

A the attack is not severe

B she should be given supplemental oxygen, but is unlikely to need a high FiO_2 to achieve normoxia

C cardiorespiratory arrest could be imminent

D her respiratory effort may be failing because she is getting tired

E she could have had a pneumothorax

Question 64

A 28-year-old man with asthma presents with an acute attack. He is very breathless and cannot complete sentences. Which of the following is the best immediate management?

A nebulised salbutamol (5 mg) driven with air

B organise chest radiograph to exclude pneumothorax

C nebulised salbutamol (5 mg) driven with high flow oxygen via reservoir bag

D nebulised salbutamol (50 mg) driven with 35% oxygen

E nebulised salbutamol (5 mg) driven with 35% oxygen

Question 65

A 72-year-old man is admitted to the coronary care unit with an acute myocardial infarction. He suffers a cardiac arrest. Basic life support is being given as you arrive. The ECG monitor reveals ventricular fibrillation (VF). The first defibrillation attempt should be made at:

A 200 J

B 400 J

C 360 J

D 20 J

E 100 J

Question 66

A 21-year-old man reports having taken an overdose of 'some tablets'. For which of the following would you NOT use activated charcoal within the first hour?

A paracetamol

B aspirin

C diazepam

D atenolol

E lithium

Infectious diseases

Alec Bonington, Carolyn Hemsley,
Michael Jacobs, Paul Klenerman and
William Lynn *(Editor)*

Infectious Diseases

Answers are on pp. 122–125.

Question 67

A 49-year-old factory worker presents unwell with fever and confusion. He is hypotensive and hypoxic. The most notable finding on clinical examination is a necrotic skin lesion on his back. He is transferred to intensive care, given supportive management and broad-spectrum antibiotics, and the surgical team consulted. The next day blood cultures flag positive with Gram-positive rods. Which two organisms should you be concerned about?

A Group A Streptococcus

B *Staphylococcus aureus*

C *Clostridium tetani*

D *Listeria monocytogenes*

E *Bacteroides fragilis*

F *Pseudomonas aeruginosa*

G *Bacillus anthracis*

H *Clostridium perfringens*

I diptheroids

J *Escherichia coli*

Question 68

This chest radiograph (Figure 5) is from a 25-year-old intravenous drug user who presented with a 10-day history of fever and a cough productive of copious amounts of green sputum. What are the two most likely aetiological agents?

A *Streptococcus pneumoniae*

B *Staphylococcus epidermidis*

C *Haemophilus influenzae*

D *Mycoplasma pneumoniae*

E *Staphylococcus aureus*

F *Legionella pneumophila*

G *Klebsiella pneumoniae*

H *Mycobacterium avium intracellulare*

I *Escherichia coli*

J *Salmonella typhi*

Question 69

A 34-year-old intravenous drug abuser presents with a persistent fever and shortness of breath. His chest radio-

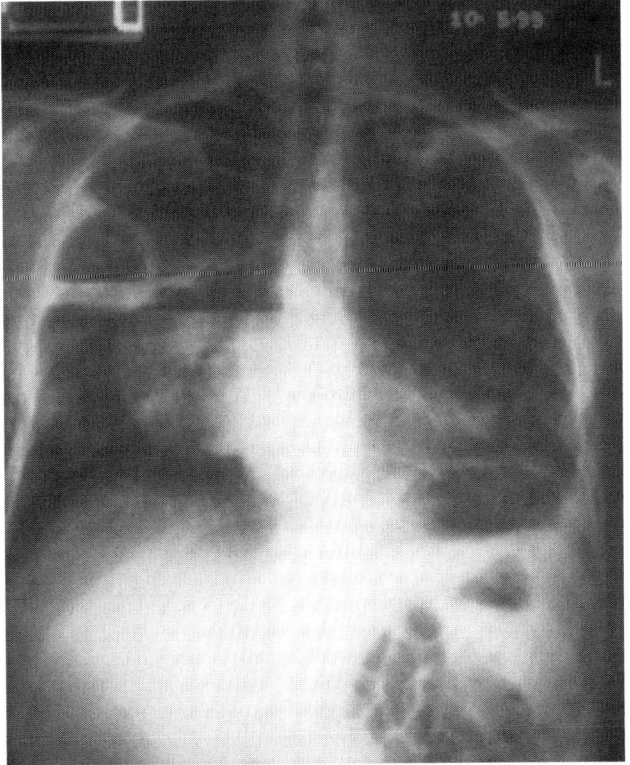

Fig. 5 Question 68.

graph shows bilateral discrete lesions. Blood cultures taken on admission flag positive after 24 hours. The Gram stain is shown (Figure 6). What is the organism (select one of options A–E) and what is the most likely underlying diagnosis (select one of options F–J)?

A *Staphylococcus aureus*

B *Streptococcus bovis*

C *Candida albicans*

D *Pneumocystis carinii*

E *Mycobacterium tuberculosis*

F HIV infection

G left-sided endocarditis

H right-sided endocarditis

I miliary tuberculosis

J pneumonia

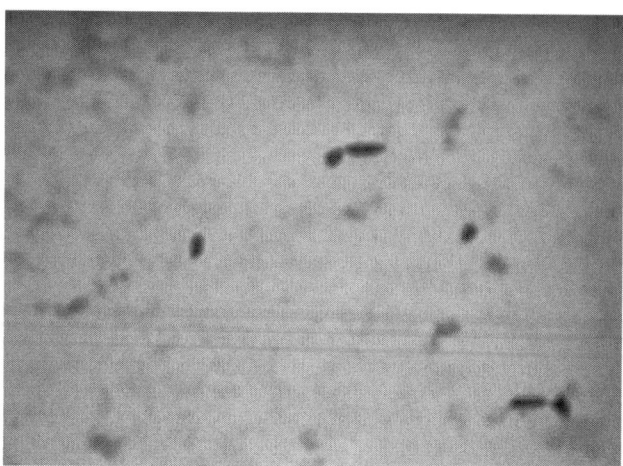

Fig. 6 Question 69.

Question 70

A 42-year-old woman has recently been diagnosed HIV positive and has a CD4 count of 180 and HIV viral load of 200 000 copies/ml. She presents with behavioural change. She is alert but withdrawn, uncommunicative, not eating and at times appears to be mute. CT brain with contrast and MRI brain show a moderate degree of cerebral atrophy but are otherwise normal. CSF analysis reveals 20 lymphocytes, protein 0.74 g/l and glucose 3.5 mmol/l (plasma 5.6 mmol/l). Which two of the following are most likely?

A CMV encephalitis

B new variant Creutzfeldt–Jacob disease

C cryptococcal meningitis

D cerebral lymphoma

E depression

F neurosyphilis

G progressive multifocal leucoencephalopathy

H cerebral toxoplasmosis

I HIV encephalopathy

J tuberculous meningitis

Question 71

A 17-year-old gay man has recently become sexually active. He presents with a 1-week history of fever, myalgia, sore throat and a macular rash. A blood film shows a reactive lymphocytosis and liver function tests are abnormal. HIV-1 antibody is negative. Which two of the following tests are most likely to provide a diagnosis?

A hepatitis C antibody

B throat, urine and stool cultures for viruses

C measurement of anti-CMV IgG

D Paul–Bunnell test

E HIV p24 antigen

F coxsackie virus serology

G HIV-2 antibody test

H blood cultures

I parvovirus B 19 IgM

J serum VDRL/TPHA

Question 72

A 48-year-old man who had been referred with deranged liver function tests attends for a follow up outpatient appointment to discuss the results of his recent tests. He is told that he has chronic hepatitis B (HBV). Which one of the following statements is correct?

A cirrhosis develops in about 20% of people with chronic hepatitis B

B all persistent HBV infection is symptomatic

C most primary infections in adults lead to persistent HBV infection

D all primary HBV infection is symptomatic

E all asymptomatic chronic HBV carriers have grossly abnormal findings on liver biopsy

Question 73

You are called to see a 78-year-old woman on an orthopae-dic ward. She fell and sustained a fractured left humerus 2 weeks previously. On admission she was noted to have an infected right venous leg ulcer and had been started on antibiotics for associated cellulitis 6 days previously. The nursing staff are concerned at a significant deterioration in her condition: she is now confused and pyrexial, and the leg ulcer has increased in size with some central necrosis and adjacent blistering. On examination some crepitus is felt. You wonder if this could be necrotising fasciitis. Which one of the following statements is correct?

A it is unlikely to be necrotising fasciitis as she is already on antibiotics

B an MRI scan maybe useful in confirming the diagnosis

C necrotising fasciitis is always caused by infection with Group A Streptococci

D crepitus does not occur in necrotising fasciitis

E bullae are unsusual in necrotising fasciitis

Question 74

A 78-year-old man has been ventilated on the Intensive Care Unit for 10 days following surgical repair of a ruptured abdominal aortic aneurysm. His respiratory function is deteriorating and it is thought that he has developed a ventilator-associated pneumonia. Which one of the following drugs might be most suitable for treatment?

A benzylpenicillin

B cefuroxime

C augmentin

D vancomycin

E piperacillin/tazobactam (Tazocin)

Question 75

A 67-year-old man with chronic renal failure (cause unknown) for which he receives regular haemodialysis treatment has been admitted to the renal ward on many occasions with access difficulties. He is now admitted with fever and malaise. Blood cultures grow a vancomycin-resistant enterococcus (VRE). Which one of the following drugs would be the most suitable treatment?

A meropenem

B linezolid

C gentamicin

D tobramycin

E co-trimoxazole (Septrin)

Question 76

A 74-year-old woman with chronic leg ulceration for which she has been admitted to hospital many times is admitted once again with fever and malaise thought to be due to infection of these ulcers. Swabs of the ulcer grow Methicillin-resistant *Staphylococcus aureus* (MRSA). Which one of the drugs listed can be used to treat this condition?

A flucloxacillin

B augmentin

C vancomycin

D cefuroxime

E meropenem

Question 77

A renal transplant patient develops fever and haematuria. Which viral infection should be considered most likely?

A polyoma virus (BK)

B Epstein-Barr virus (EBV)

C herpes simplex virus (HSV)

D varicella zoster (VZV)

E human herpes virus6 (HHV-6).

Question 78

A woman who is 36 weeks pregnant presents with chickenpox. How should she be treated?

A varicella-zoster immune globulin

B steroids

C aciclovir

D painkillers only

E immediate delivery of the child

Question 79

An intubated patient on the Intensive Care Unit for 8 days following a road traffic accident has a persistent fever and some lung shadowing. Which of the following organisms is most likely to be involved?

A *Streptococcus pneumoniae*

B *Staphylococcus epidermidis*

C *Staphylococcus aureus*

D *Pseudomonas aeruginosa*

E *Legionella pneumophila*

Question 80

A 28-year-old woman has noticed this blistering eruption appear over her body every 2–3 months for the last year (see Figure 7). On each occasion she has had

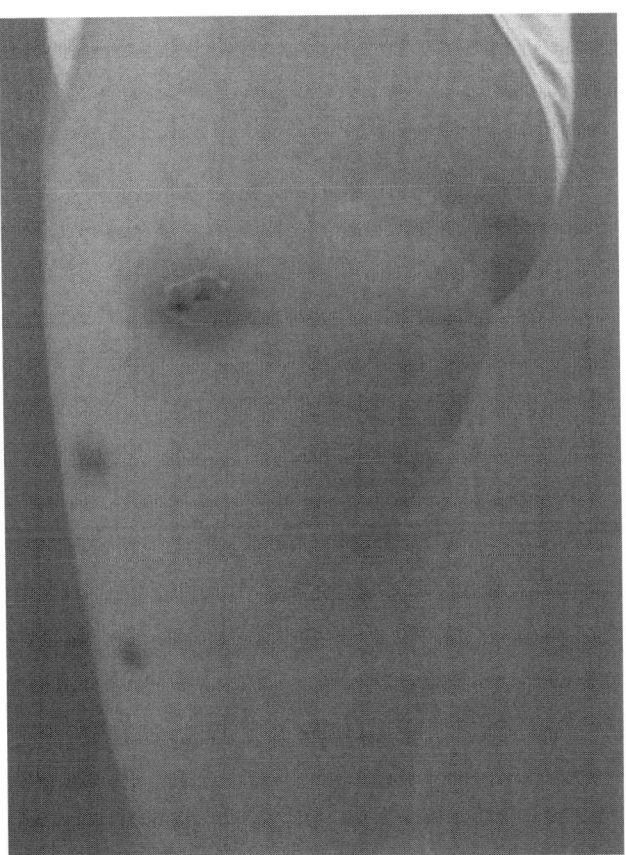

Fig. 7 Question 80.

symptoms of genital soreness and has taken some potassium citrate and cranberry juice. What is the most likely diagnosis?

A fixed drug eruption

B erythema multiforme

C disseminated gonococcal disease

D bullous pemphigus

E urticaria

Question 81

A 25-year-old woman complains of an increasing offensive vaginal discharge over the last 2 weeks. She is feeling feverish and has lower abdominal pains. She is not sexually active and has had a sexual health screen after she finished her last relationship some 3 months ago when a cervical erosion was noted. She has never had a sexually transmitted infection. She is on no medication and her last normal menstrual period was 17 days ago. She discontinued her oral contraceptive some 4 weeks ago. What is the most likely diagnosis?

A candidal infection

B *Neisseria gonorrhoeae* infection

C cervical malignancy

D retained foreign body in the vagina

E pregnancy

Question 82

A patient reports that he is allergic to erythromycin. Which one of the following would you NOT usually accept as being compatible with an allergic reaction?

A fever

B widespread rash

C shortness of breath

D diarrhoea

E localized skin eruption

Question 83

An 89-year-old man presents to casualty with a fever and a several week history of headache. On examination he is confused, has neck stiffness and a right seventh cranial nerve palsy. He has no visible rash. A lumbar puncture reveals CSF Protein 4.0 g/l, Glucose 1.2 mmol/l (plasma glucose 4.6 mmol/l), and on microscopy 300 white cells/μl, predominantly lymphocytes. Serum VDRL is positive and TPHA is negative. The most likely diagnosis is:

A viral meningitis

B neurosyphilis

C herpes simplex encephalitis

D tuberculous meningitis

E *Listeria* meningitis

Question 84

A 32-year-old woman presents with community-acquired pneumonia. She is very unwell, but reports that she is 'allergic to penicillin', having had an anaphylactic reaction after treatment of a urinary tract infection several years ago. You would give her:

A cefotaxime 2 g six-hourly and erythromycin 1 g six-hourly, both intravenously

B erythromicin 500 mg six-hourly orally

C amoxicillin 250 mg eight-hourly and clarithromycin 250 mg twice daily, both orally

D erythromycin 1 g six-hourly intravenously

E ciprofloxacin 500 mg twice daily orally

Question 85

A 77-year-old man presents with sudden onset of weakness of his right arm on a background of a 3-week history of thoracolumbar backpain, weight loss, fever and night sweats. Blood tests show haemoglobin 9.8 g/dL, white cell count (WCC) 12.0×10^9/l, platelets 450×10^9/l, erythrocyte sedimentation rate (ESR) 110 mm/hr, creatinine 180 μmol/L. Stick testing of his urine reveals microscopic haematuria. What is the most likely diagnosis?

A spinal osteomyelitis

B myeloma

C infective endocarditis

D mycobacterium tuberculosis infection

E tertiary syphilis

Question 86

A 48-year-old man presents on the medical take with right lower lobe pneumonia. In the acute assessment of an adult with community-acquired pneumonia which one of the following is NOT of prognostic importance?

A urea > 7 mmol/l

B confusional state

C PaO_2 < 10 kPa

D respiratory rate > 30/min

E diastolic BP < 60 mmHg

Question 87

A 57-year-old woman develops a fever 7 days post bone marrow transplantation. She is placed empirically on broad-spectrum antibiotics but remains febrile. On the 11th day she develops a few painless, red, papular lesions on her trunk and lower limbs. What is the likely cause of these lesions?

A candidal infection

B staphylococcal infection

C aspergillus infection

D graft versus host disease

E recurrence of her haematological disease

Question 88

A 26-year-old woman presents with a short history of confusion, diarrhoea and breathlessness. On examination she is pyrexial at 38.5°C, pulse 120/min, BP 80/60 mmHg and respiratory rate 26/min. She has a faint blanching macular rash across the trunk. She is disorientated without meningism. Which of the following diagnoses is most likely?

A *Salmonella enteritidis* infection

B pneumococcal meningitis

C anaphylaxis

D N-methyl-3,4-methylenedioxymethamphetamine ('Ecstasy') overdose

E toxic shock syndrome

Question 89

A 30-year-old man presents with diplopia, dysphagia and dysarthria. After 12 hours he has weakness of his arms but remains afebrile and is not confused. Over the next 12 hours he develops respiratory failure and requires artificial ventilation. What is the likely diagnosis?

A tetanus

B diphtheria

C botulism

D strychnine poisoning

E rabies

Question 90

A 38-year-old man presents with breathlessness and cough. He is unwell, with high fever, and has signs of consolidation in his right lower lobe. The most likely pathogen is:

A legionella

B *Neisseria meningitidis*

C *Streptococcus pneumoniae*

D HIV

E *Staphylococcus aureus*

Question 91

An HIV-positive patient presents with abdominal bloating and discomfort. He is afebrile, with blood pressure 110/60 mmHg, pulse 98/min, respiratory rate 24/min. The chest is clear, heart sounds normal, but palpation reveals some right upper quadrant tenderness. Blood tests show Na 141 mmol/L, K 3.9 mmol/L, urea 7.2 mmol/L, creatinine 111 μmol/L, bilirubin 48 μmol/L, alkaline phosphatase 500 IU/L, gamma-glutamyl transpeptidase (GGT) 220 IU/L, alanine aminotransferase (ALT) 80 IU/L. Arterial blood gases (breathing air) are pH 7.28, PaO_2 12.0 kPa, PCO_2 3.2 kPa, base excess –11.9. A chest radiograph is normal. The CD4 count is 180 cells/mL and HIV viral load is undetectable. What is the most likely diagnosis?

A *Pneumocystis carinii* pneumonia

B myocardial infarction

C *Mycobacterium avium* infection

D lactic acidosis

E hepatitis C infection

Dermatology

Karen Harman *(Editor)*, Graham Ogg and
Natalie M Stone

Dermatology

Answers are on pp. 125–126.

Question 92
A 48-year-old man developed a chronic rash on his forehead, nose, cheeks and chin (see Figure 8). What is the likely diagnosis?

A rosacea
B acne
C atopic eczema
D dermatomyositis
E photosensitive eczema

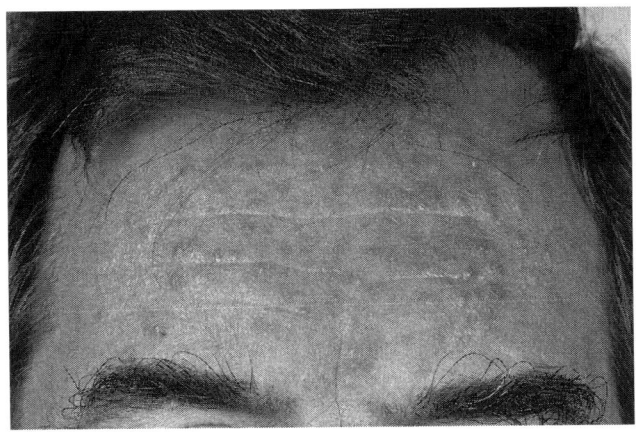

Fig. 8 Question 92.

Question 93
A 20-year-old trainee hairdresser develops an intensely itchy, erythematous scaly rash on her hands. The two most common diagnoses would be:

A irritant hand dermatitis
B contact allergic dermatitis
C psoriasis
D lichen planus
E urticaria
F porphyria
G mycosis fungoides
H erythema multiforme
I bullous pemphigoid
J hand, foot and mouth disease

Question 94
A 28-year-old woman presents with painful lumps on her legs (see Figure 9). What are the two most likely diagnoses?

A Sezary syndrome
B erythema nodosum
C nodular vasculitis
D necrobiosis lipoidica
E mycosis fungoides
F discoid lupus erythematosus
G contact dermatitis
H pre-tibial myxoedema
I insect bites
J psoriasis

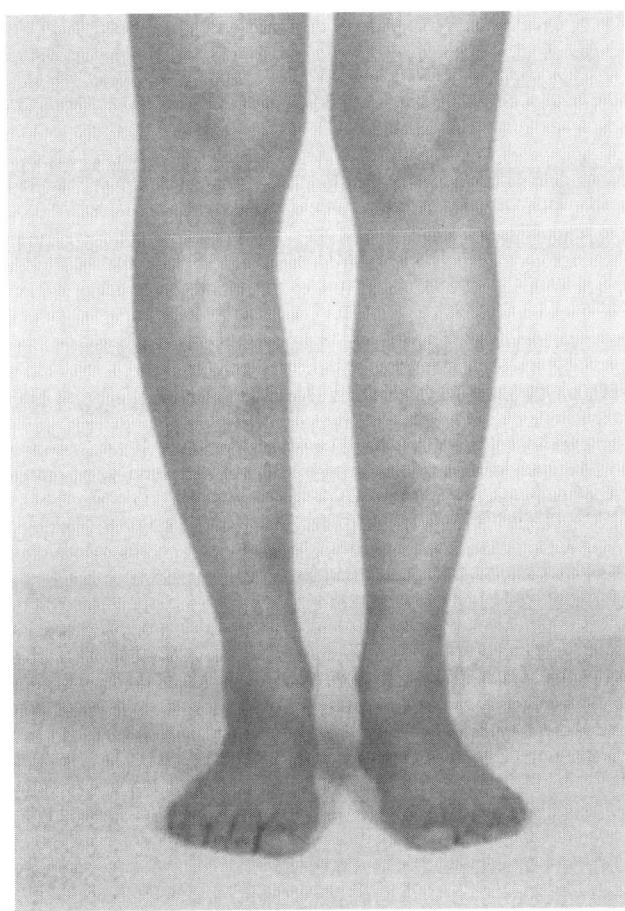

Fig. 9 Question 94.

Question 95

A 16-year-old girl presents with an itchy rash 3 days after arriving on holiday in the Mediterranean. Examination reveals an erythematous papular rash over the arms and trunk, sparing sites under her swimming costume and sparing her face and hands. What is the most likely diagnosis?

A systemic lupus erythematosus
B polymorphic light eruption
C photoallergic contact dermatitis
D scabies
E xeroderma pigmentosum

Question 96

A 30-year-old woman presents with a 5-year history of flushing of her facial skin and a spotty rash. Examination reveals a pustular rash on the cheeks with no comedones. What is the most likely diagnosis?

A rosacea
B acne vulgaris
C carcinoid syndrome
D systemic lupus erythematosus (SLE)
E allergic contact dermatitis

Question 97

A 17-year-old girl has developed an eczematous patch just below her umbilicus, thought to be due to allergy to a stud fastener in her jeans. Which one of the following statements is true regarding allergic contact dermatitis to nickel?

A it is diagnosed by prick testing
B it is a type 3 allergic reaction
C it affects males and females equally
D it occurs more commonly in atopic patients
E it can be caused by wearing gold jewellery

Question 98

A 60-year-old cleaner presents with a rash on both hands. An irritant hand dermatitis is suspected. Which one of the following statements is true regarding this condition?

A it classically causes a finger tip dermatitis
B it is diagnosed by patch testing
C it is more common in atopic patients
D it can be differentiated from allergic contact dermatitis histologically
E it should not be treated with topical steroids

Question 99

A 58-year-old man presents with a scaly rash. You consider the diagnosis of psoriasis. Which one of the following statements is true of this condition?

A psoriasis shows the Koebner phenomenon
B nail involvement in psoriasis is rare
C guttate psoriasis is the commonest form
D sterile pustules are frequently seen within lesions
E intense pruritus is a typical symptom

Haematology

Kristian M Bowles, David W Galvani *(Editor)*
and Bronwen E Shaw

Haematology

Answers are on pp. 126–128.

Question 100

A 39-year-old factory worker is seen in clinic with a 4-week history of increasing fatigue and a swelling in his neck (see Figure 10). His blood count is reported as follows: haemoglobin 8.7 g/dl, white cell count 12.2×10^9/l (neutrophils 3.0×10^9/l) and platelets 97×10^9/l. His plasma viscosity is raised at 2.9 kPa/s, and his creatinine is also elevated at 256 μmol/l. A fine needle aspiration of the neck swelling produces cellular material (see Figure 11). The most likely diagnosis is:

A acute lymphoblastic leukaemia

B acute myeloid leukaemia

C lymphoma

D myeloma

E Epstein Barr Virus infection

Question 101

A 73-year-old man had been treated for myeloma with 6 cycles of chemotherapy, each cycle consisting of four days of continuous intravenous chemotherapy given at monthly

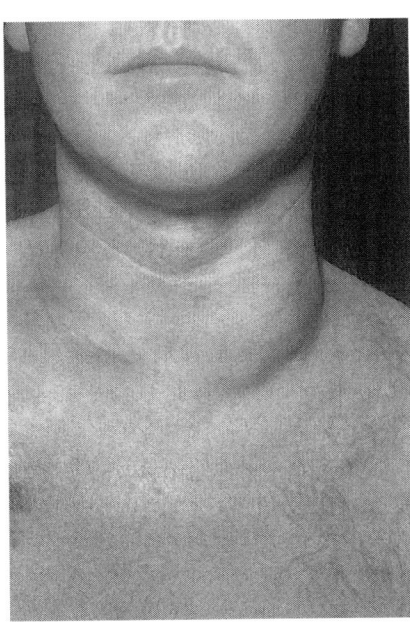

Fig. 10 Question 100.

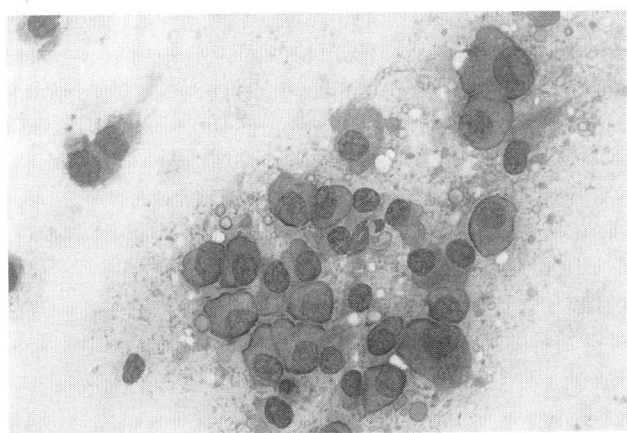

Fig. 11 Question 100.

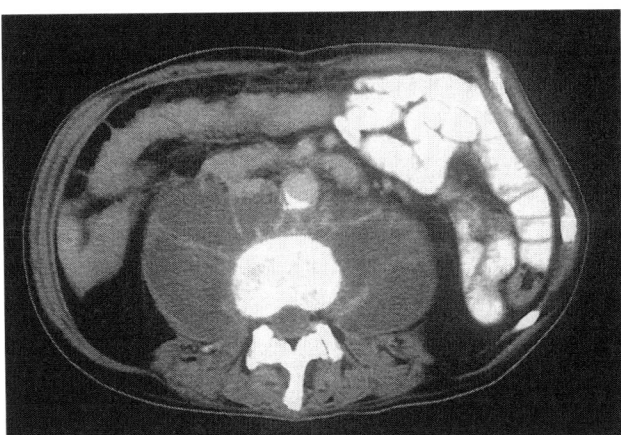

Fig. 12 Question 101.

intervals via a Hickman line. He had suffered from several episodes of pyrexia which settled with broad spectrum antimicrobials.

He is now admitted with lower abdominal pain and difficulty walking. There are no clear-cut neurological signs, but he finds it difficult to move his legs because of pain.

His blood count shows haemoglobin 9.1 g/dl, white cell count 15.9×10^9/l (neutrophils 7.0×10^9/l) and platelets 110×10^9/l. A CT scan of his abdomen is performed (see Figure 12). The most likely diagnosis is:

A psoas abscesses

B myelomatous soft tissue mass around spine

C osteomyelitis of spine

D myelomatous destruction of vertebrae

E rupture of abdominal aorta

Question 102

A 24-year-old woman presented with purpura (see Figure 13). She had similar appearances of purpura on the other leg and the flexor aspects of the forearms. Her blood count is as follows: haemoglobin 12.1 g/dl, mean corpuscular volume 81 fl, white cell count $10 \times 10^9/l$ and platelets $187 \times 10^9/l$. A full clotting screen was normal. What is the most likely diagnosis?

A idiopathic thrombocytopenic purpura

B factitious purpura

C Henoch-Schönlein purpura

D mixed essential cryoglobulinaemia

E purpura fulminans

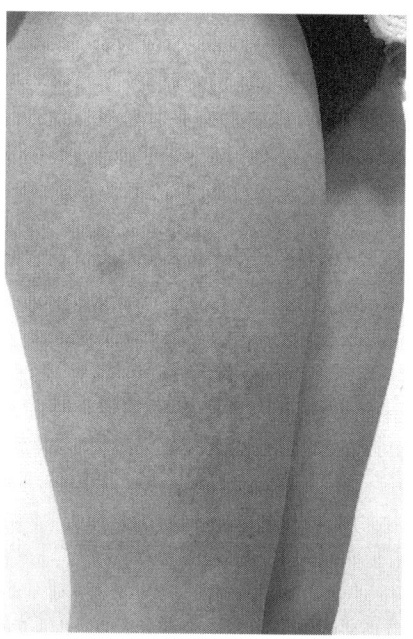

Fig. 13 Question 102.

Question 103

A 31-year-old woman is admitted as an emergency, having been found unconscious at home by her mother, who said that over the past few days she had suffered from 'flu like symptoms, with high fever and confusion in the last 24 hours. She is febrile, with temperature 38.7°C, pulse 110/min, respiratory rate 14/min and BP 190/110 mmHg. Her blood count is as follows: haemoglobin 9.7 g/dl, white cell count $15 \times 10^9/l$ (neutrophils $11 \times 10^9/l$) and platelets

$16 \times 10^9/l$. A full clotting screen is normal. Figure 14 shows her blood film. What is the most likely diagnosis?

A sickle cell anaemia—neurological crisis

B falciparum malaria

C thrombotic thrombocytopenic purpura

D malignant hypertension

E acute myeloid leukaemia

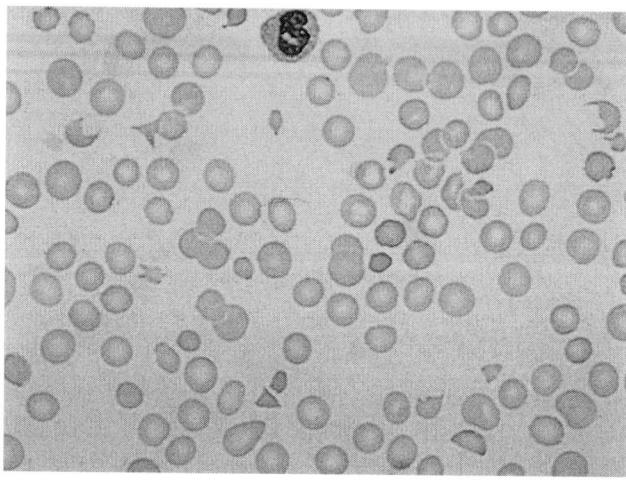

Fig. 14 Question 103.

Question 104

A 72-year-old man with primary proliferative polycythaemia has had regular venesections for seven years to control his polycythaemia. Figure 15 shows the appearance of his thumbnails. What is the most likely reason for these appearances?

A chronic liver disease

B intermittent episodes of ill health

C psoriasis

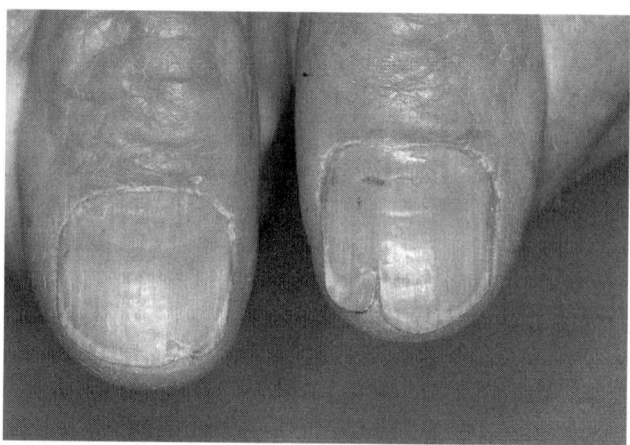

Fig. 15 Question 104.

D iron deficiency

E chronic lung disease

Question 105

A 28-year-old man has a splenectomy after a road traffic accident. Which one of the treatment strategies listed is NOT required?

A meningococcal vaccination

B *Haemophilus influenzae* vaccination

C prophylactic antibiotics with penicillin V or erythromycin

D polyvalent pneumococcal vaccination

E hepatitis B vaccination

Question 106

A 44-year-old man vomited some blood, but this settled down and he did not seek a medical opinion, thinking that it was due to 'something that he had eaten.' The next day he had a nose bleed and was sent to the medical admissions unit by his general practitioner. On examination he had an extensive purpuric rash over the trunk and on direct questioning said that he had been bruising very easily for the last week or so. His full blood count showed severe thrombocytopenia with a platelet count of $2 \times 10^9/l$. A bone marrow examination showed normal numbers of megakaryocytes and a diagnosis of idiopathic thrombocytopenic purpura was made. What is the most appropriate treatment for him?

A oral prednisolone 60 mg

B pulsed intravenous methyl prednisolone at a dose of 1 g

C intravenous immunoglobulin

D platelet transfusions

E intravenous thrombopoietin infusion

Question 107

A 38-year-old man has had two deep venous thromboses in the absence of any recognised precipitating events. You ask the haematology laboratory to screen for causes of a thrombophilic state. Which one of the following conditions will they NOT look for?

A protein C deficiency

B protein S deficiency

C antithrombin III deficiency

D factor VIII deficiency

E lupus anticoagulant

Question 108

A 55-year-old woman presents with tiredness. She had been given a diagnosis of rheumatoid arthritis at the age of 35, but has been fit and well for many years, without any joint problems. Her full blood count is as follows: Hb 9.3 g/dl, MVC 85 fl, MCH 28 pg, white blood cell count normal, platelet count normal. Which one of the following statements is correct?

A sideroblastic anaemia is a likely diagnosis

B Felty's syndrome is a likely diagnosis

C acute blood loss is likely

D anaemia of chronic disorders is the most likely diagnosis

E a normal ferritin excludes iron deficiency as a cause of her anaemia

Question 109

A tall thin 18-year-old man with sickle cell disease presents to the Accident and Emergency department with a 36-hour history of cough, fever, breathlessness and pleuritic chest pain. The most likely diagnosis is:

A pulmonary embolism

B myocardial infarction

C pneumococcal pneumonia

D pneumothorax

E acute chest syndrome

Question 110

A 49-year-old man presents with melaena of a week's duration. On investigation his platelet count is found to be elevated. Which of the following is the most likely cause of the thrombocytosis?

A blood loss

B chronic myeloid leukaemia

C infection

D essential thrombocythaemia

E inflammatory bowel disease

Question 111

A previously well 34-year-old woman (gravida II, para II) who is 24 weeks pregnant presents with a low platelet count of $84 \times 10^9/L$. She is asymptomatic and experienced similar problems in her last pregnancy, following which she gave birth to a normal healthy boy. She denies any previous medical history or family history of a blood disorder. Which one of the following statements is true?

A a bone marrow aspirate will confirm chronic idiopathic thrombocytopenic purpura (ITP)

B a Caesarian section should be the preferred delivery method

C the baby has a 10% risk of intracranial bleed

D no investigations are required and platelets should normalise post partum

E platelet associated immunoglobulins will be high

Question 112

A 24-year-old woman presents to the Accident and Emergency department with a history of a painless swelling in her neck. She is otherwise well. What is the most likely diagnosis from the following list?

A acute leukaemia

B infectious mononucleosis

C non-Hodgkin's lymphoma

D HIV seroconversion illness

E Hodgkin's disease

Oncology

Mark Bower *(Editor)* and Graham G Dark

Oncology

Answers are on pp. 128–130.

Question 113
A 78-year-old man presents with a spot on his forehead that has been gradually getting bigger over about 6 months (see Figure 16). The most likely diagnosis is:

A basal cell carcinoma

B squamous cell carcinoma

C amelanotic melanoma

D viral wart

E psoriatic plaque

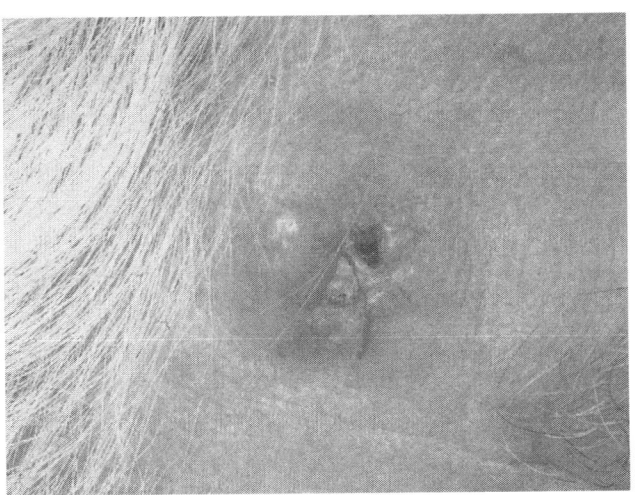

Fig. 16 Question 113.

Question 114
A 28-year-old teacher was admitted with a three-week history of breathlessness, non-productive cough, intermittent low-grade fever, fatigue and malaise. Ten months previously he had been diagnosed with metastatic testicular teratoma. After treatment with orchidectomy and four cycles of BEP (bleomycin, etoposide and cisplatin), abdominal CT scan showed no evidence of tumour. On admission he was breathless on minimal exertion and there were end-inspiratory crackles throughout both lungs. His chest radiograph is shown (see Figure 17). The most likely diagnosis is:

A bronchopneumonia

B pulmonary oedema

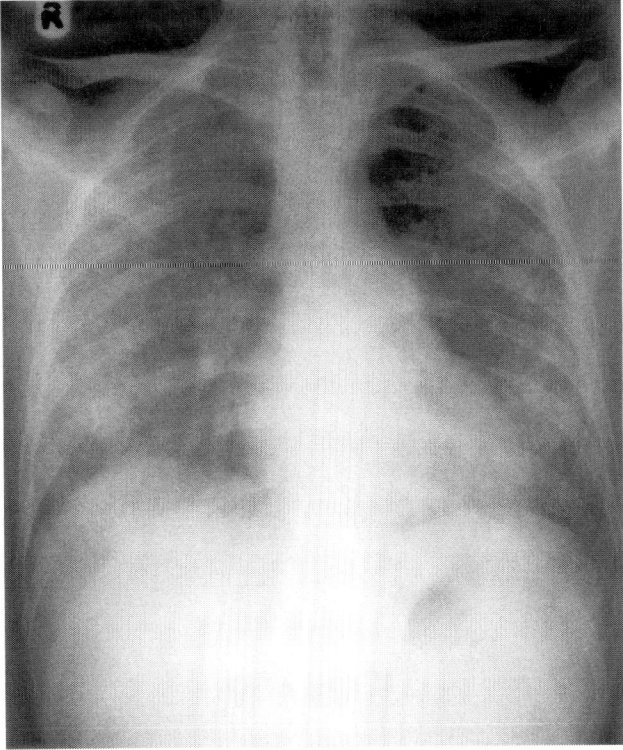

Fig. 17 Question 114.

C *Pneumocystis carinii* pneumonia

D metastatic teratoma

E bleomycin toxicity

Question 115
A 68-year-old man presents with rectal bleeding and is found to have carcinoma of the rectum. Investigation shows no evidence of distant metastases. Which two of the following are accepted initial treatment regimens?

A surgical resection

B radiotherapy followed by surgical resection

C chemotherapy followed by surgical resection

D radiotherapy and chemotherapy followed by surgical resection

E surgical resection followed by radiotherapy depending on findings at operation

F surgical resection followed by chemotherapy depending on findings at operation

G surgical resection followed by radiotherapy and chemotherapy depending on findings at operation

H radiotherapy

I chemotherapy

J watchful waiting

Question 116

A 35-year-old woman presents with weight loss and a mass of lymph nodes at the base of her neck. Histology of the nodes revealed a poorly differentiated squamous cell carcinoma. Aside from the nodes, examination of the head and neck is normal, as is specialist ENT examination and CT scan of the head and neck. What are the two most likely sites for the primary?

A breast

B oesophageal

C colon

D ovary

E kidney

F skin

G anus

H cervical

I lung

J liver

Question 117

A 45-year-old woman has recently been diagnosed with malignant mesothelioma. Which of the following two are not useful as prognostic factors in mesothelioma

A poor performance status

B male gender

C non-epithelial histology

D low haemoglobin

E high platelet count

F high lactate dehydrogenase (LDH)

G high white blood count

H history of asbestos exposure

I history of cigarette smoking

J weight loss

Question 118

A 58-year-old woman presents with left chest wall pain after a coughing fit. Eight years ago she had a mastectomy, adjuvant chemotherapy and endocrine therapy and chest wall radiotherapy of a T2N1 cancer of the left breast. Her bone scan now shows a solitary hot spot in the anterior left 5th rib. Which one of the following statements is INCORRECT?

A a follow-up bone scan in 6 months is indicated

B the hot spot is likely to be a fracture from radiation induced osteoporosis

C the hot spot is likely to be a radiation induced sarcoma

D the hot spot is likely to be a fracture from metastatic disease

E a raised alkaline phosphatase would be helpful in the differential diagnosis

Question 119

A 28-year-old woman reports that several of her family members have died of breast cancer, including her mother at age 43, her maternal aunt at age 62 and her maternal grandmother at age 65. What is the probability that she will develop breast cancer?

A 5%

B 10%

C 20%

D 40%

E 80%

Question 120

A 49-year-old man presents to his general practitioner with a history of chronic intermittent diarrhoea. On examination he has a flushed appearance and facial telangiectasia. He has a heart murmur and hepatomegaly that is nodular and firm. Laboratory results are as follows: Na 130 mmol/l, K 2.5 mmol/l, Urea 12.2 mmol/l, Creatinine 119 µmol/l, Ca 2.4 mmol/l, albumin 29 g/l, ALT 27 IU/l. Which single test may assist in confirming the diagnosis?

A serum carcinoembryonic antigen (CEA)

B serum tumour marker, CA 19-9

C 24 hour urinary 5-hydroxyindoleacetic acid

D 24 hour urinay vanillylmandelic acid

E serum catecholamines

Question 121

A 55-year-old man presents with haematuria, loin swelling and discomfort. A CT scan shows a large renal mass with tumour in the renal vein but not the inferior vena cava, and bilateral small lung metastases. What is the most appropriate treatment option?

A immunotherapy

B radical nephrectomy and medroxyprogesterone acetate

C chemotherapy

D renal artery embolisation and immunotherapy

E radical nephrectomy and immunotherapy

Question 122

A 65-year-old woman with increasing abdominal pain is found to have a pelvic mass on physical examination. After appropriate staging studies she undergoes a laparotomy and is found to have serous carcinoma of the ovary with involvement of one ovary and several omental implants. She then undergoes a hysterectomy, bilateral salpingo-oophorectomy, liver biopsy, omentectomy, cytological examination of abdominal washings, and extensive inspection. All evidence of disease is removed. Assuming generally good health, an uneventful postoperative recovery, and lack of proximity to a centre performing clinical trials, what is the most appropriate management?

A no further therapy
B combination chemotherapy
C combination chemotherapy only if serum CA125 level is elevated
D intraperitoneal chemotherapy
E whole abdominal radiation therapy

Question 123

A 75-year-old man with a 30-pack year cigarette smoking history complains of continuous right shoulder pain, a persistent cough and weight loss. His chest radiograph shows a right apical shadow. On examination you note that he is clubbed, has a small right pupil and a right-sided ptosis. What is the most likely diagnosis?

A small cell lung cancer
B squamous cell carcinoma
C bronchoalveolar carcinoma of the lung
D adenocarcinoma of the left lung
E bronchial carcinoid

Question 124

A 76-year-old woman presents with haemoptysis and clubbing. A diagnosis of lung cancer is made. Which is the most likely histological subtype?

A small cell lung cancer
B bronchoalveolar carcinoma
C carcinoid
D squamous cell lung cancer
E adenocarcinoma

Question 125

A 28-year-old woman presents with an enlarging mole on her calf. Excision biopsy shows a superficial spreading melanoma of 0.5 mm thickness. Subsequent treatment should be:

A wide excision and adjuvant immunotherapy
B wide excision with 1 cm margin
C wide excision and sentinel node biopsy
D wide excision and elective inguinal node dissection
E wide excision with 5 cm margin

Question 126

A patient with lymphoma excretes 1.5 g urinary protein/day but has a negative urinary dipstick test for protein. The reason for this seeming inconsistency is:

A dipsticks preferentially detect albumin rather than immunoglobulin because albumin is negatively charged
B the molecular weight of the excreted protein is too low to be detected by dipsticks
C Tamm-Horsfall proteins block the reaction of the secreted protein and the dipstick
D the urine is not sufficiently concentrated
E dipsticks only recognise heavy chain sequences

Question 127

Following chemotherapy a patient develops symmetrical paraesthesia and sensory loss over the toes of both feet. Which one of the following cytotoxics is LEAST likely to cause this side effect?

A vincristine
B doxorubicin
C docetaxel
D cisplatin
E paclitaxel

Cardiology

Peter E Glennon, Catherine EG Head,
Paul R Roberts *(Editor)* and
Hamish A Walker

Cardiology

Answers are on pp. 130–132.

Question 128

A 28-year-old woman becomes dizzy with a feeling of heaviness in the chest when jogging with a friend. She stops, sits down, and over a few minutes she improves so that she can walk home. The friend brings her to the Accident and Emergency department, where you are asked to assess her. Aside from dizziness and heaviness she was not aware of any other symptoms and she has not had the problem before. She has no significant past medical history and takes the oral contraceptive pill as her only regular medication. Physical examination is normal. Her ECG is shown (see Figure 18). What is the most likely diagnosis?

A acute myocardial infarction

B pulmonary embolism

C paroxysmal atrial fibrillation

D Wolff-Parkinson-White syndrome

E acute pericarditis

Question 129

A 58-year-old man presents with severe ischaemic chest pain. His ECG is shown (see Figure 19). Which is the best description of the ECG?

A acute anterior myocardial infarction

B acute anterolateral myocardial infarction

C acute anterolateral myocardial infarction with ventricular ectopics

D acute anterior myocardial infarction with ventricular ectopics

E acute anterolateral myocardial infarction with posterior extension

Question 130

A 63-year-old man with Marfan's syndrome presents with chest pain and is found to have an acute aortic dissection. Which two of the following cardiac conditions are associated with Marfan's?

A atrial myxoma

B mitral stenosis

C pulmonary regurgitation

D ventricular tachycardia

E atrial septal defect

F ventricular septal defect

G cardiac amyloid

H sarcoidosis

I mitral valve prolapse

J aortic stenosis

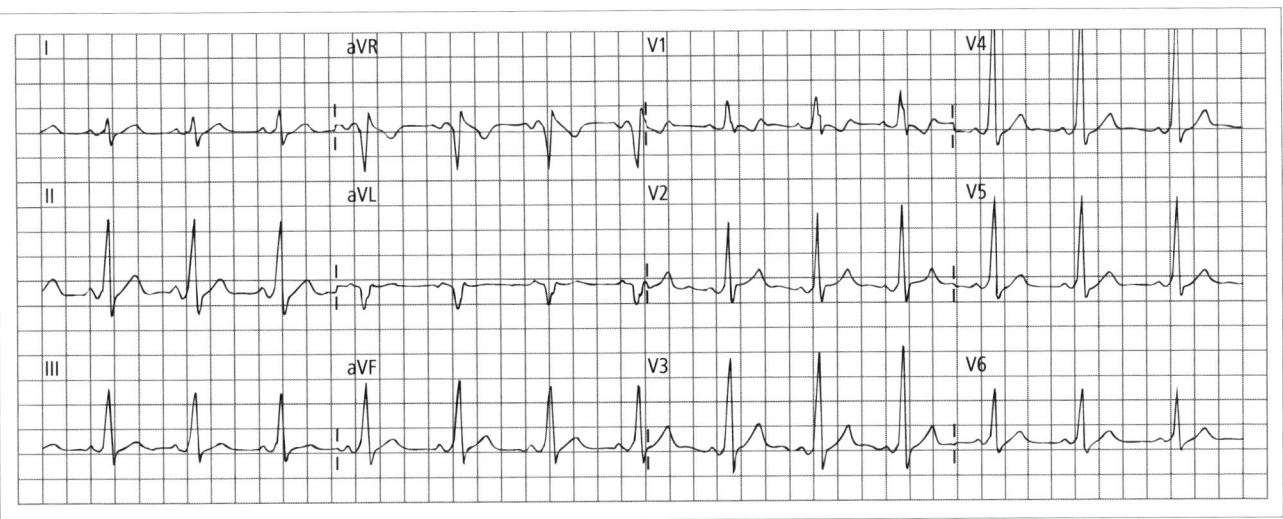

Fig. 18 Question 128.

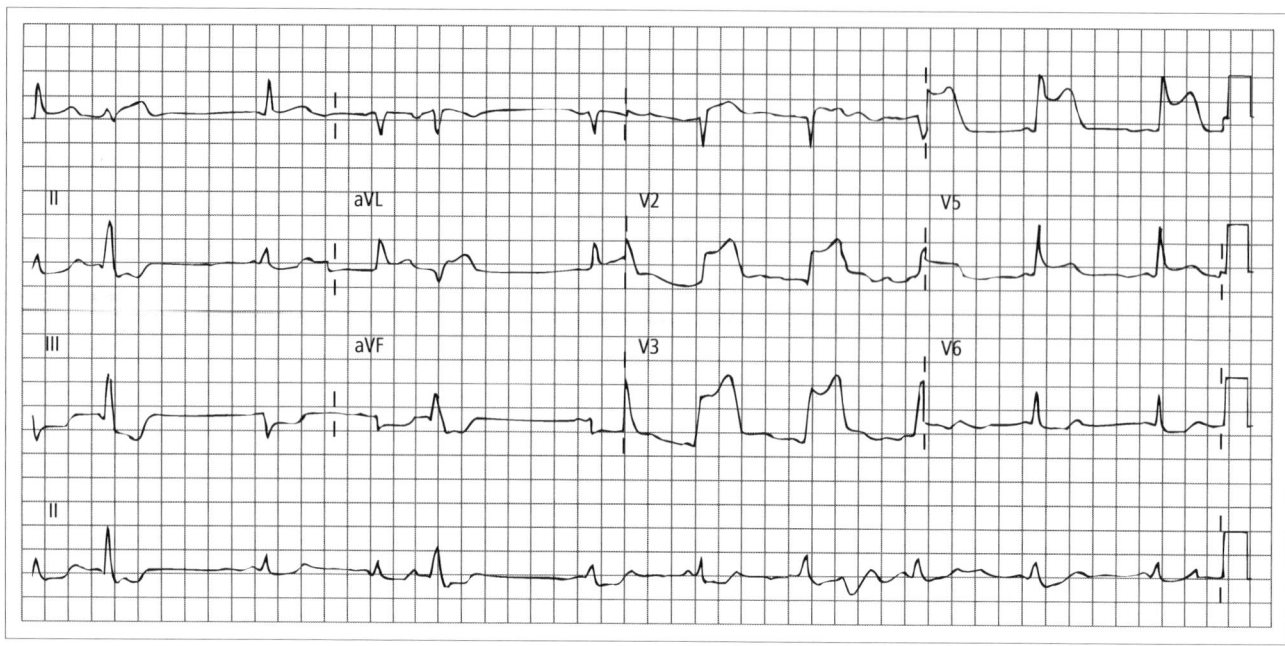

Fig. 19 Question 129.

Question 131

A 77-year-old man presents with 5 hours of chest pain at rest. He had undergone stenting to his left anterior descending artery 4 years previously. ECG shows inferior T-wave inversion, with ventricular ectopics. His troponin T is elevated at 0.4. He is already taking aspirin. Which two of the following would be considered appropriate initial therapeutic interventions?

A amiodarone
B change aspirin to clopidogrel
C coronary artery bypass grafting
D digoxin
E flecainide
F Glycoprotein IIb/IIa receptor blocker
G percutaneous coronary intervention
H dipyridamole (modified release)
I prophylactic dose of low molecular weight heparin
J thrombolysis

Question 132

A 48-year-old man is found to have a blood pressure of 176/112 mmHg when he attends his general practitioner for a 'new patient check-up'. He takes occasional anxiolytics for anxiety, but his past medical history is otherwise unremarkable. Physical examination is normal, excepting for obesity (BMI 32). A 'routine' biochemical screen is normal, excepting for potassium 3.3 mmol/l. The two most likely causes of his hypertension are:

A renal hypertension
B hypothyroidism
C renovascular hypertension
D Cushing's syndrome
E primary hyperaldosteronism (Conn's syndrome)
F acromegaly
G essential hypertension
H isolated clinic ('white coat') hypertension
I phaeochromocytoma
J coarctation of the aorta

Question 133

A 60-year-old man is being investigated for chest pain and undergoes exercise tolerance testing. Which of the following features is associated with a worse prognosis?

A increased heart rate with exercise
B ventricular tachycardia
C increase in blood pressure with exercise
D rapid resolution of heart rate in recovery
E absence of symptoms during exercise

Question 134

A 45-year-old man with dilated cardiomyopathy is being considered for cardiac transplantation. Which of the following is generally deemed to be a contraindication to cardiac transplantation?

A any previous cancer

B pulmonary artery wedge pressure <20 mmHg

C creatinine clearance <50 ml min⁻¹

D previous alcoholism

E hypertension

Question 135

A patient with documented systolic dysfunction has permanent atrial fibrillation. His resting heart rate is 100 and systolic blood pressure 120 mmHg; there is no evidence of fluid retention. Creatinine is normal and he is already receiving appropriate doses of furosemide and angiotensin-converting-enzyme (ACE) inhibitor. Which of the following would be the next therapy?

A amiodarone

B carvidolol

C DC cardioversion

D digoxin

E metoprolol

Question 136

A 78-year-old man with known ischaemic heart disease and congestive cardiac failure is admitted as an emergency with severe pulmonary oedema. He is sitting with his legs over the side of the casualty trolley and gasping. He has smoked 20 cigarettes per day for many years. What is the first treatment he should receive?

A furosemide 40 mg intravenously

B high flow oxygen via reservoir bag

C 35% oxygen

D diamorphine 2.5 mg intravenously, with anti-emetic

E isosorbide dinitrate by intravenous infusion at dose titrated against blood pressure

Question 137

A 60-year-old woman develops hypotension and a new systolic murmur 36 hours after being successfully thrombolysed for an anterior myocardial infarction. Which of the following statements is correct?

A acute mitral incompetence due to rupture of the posterior papillary muscle is the most likely diagnosis

B acute mitral incompetence due to rupture of the anterior papillary muscle is the most likely diagnosis

C a basal ventricular septal defect (VSD) is the most likely diagnosis

D an apical ventricular septal defect is the most likely diagnosis

E the systolic murmur is likely to be due to mitral valve prolapse

Question 138

A 70-year-old woman presents with 8 hours of chest pain. Her pulse rate is 40/minute and blood pressure 105/85. The ECG shows complete heart block, ST segment elevation and Q waves in leads II, III and AVF. Which of the following statements is correct?

A atropine should be given immediately

B an isoprenaline infusion should be set up immediately

C thrombolysis should be given immediately

D thrombolysis should be avoided because she has completed her myocardial infarction

E thrombolysis should be avoided because she may require a temporary pacing wire

Question 139

A 68-year-old man is admitted to the coronary care unit and thrombolysed for an inferior myocardial infarction. He makes an uneventful recovery. His total serum cholesterol on the admission blood test is 4.8 mmol/L. What action should be taken?

A he should be reassured that his cholesterol is normal

B he should have a repeat fasting serum cholesterol measured before discharge from hospital

C he should receive dietary advice and have his serum cholesterol measured in 3 month's time

D he should be started on an HMG Coenzyme A inhibitor

E a full lipid profile should be obtained and lipid lowering drug treatment started if his LDL fraction is >3.5 mmol/L and his HDL is <1.0 mmol/L

Question 140

A 20-year-old female student presents with central chest pain after four days of a 'flu-like illness. She has no significant past medical history and takes the oral contraceptive pill as her only regular medication. The most likely diagnosis is:

A acute viral pericarditis

B gastro-oesophageal reflux

C acute myocardial infarction

D systemic lupus erythematosus

E pulmonary embolism

Question 141

A 28-year-old woman presents with breathlessness and pleuritic chest pain. Which of the following test results is more than 90% specific for excluding pulmonary embolism (PE) in a patient presenting with a high clinical probability of the diagnosis?

A negative D-dimer

B normal lung perfusion on V/Q scan

C no evidence of PE on spiral CT

D normal chest radiograph and arterial blood gases

E no evidence of deep vein thrombosis (DVT) on lower limb venography

Question 142

A 59-year-old man with moderate chronic obstructive lung disease is admitted breathless following an episode of syncope while shopping. There is no previous history of syncope. Past history includes multiple stab ligations for bilateral varicose veins four weeks previously and open cholecystectomy 10 years before. On examination he is breathless at rest, apyrexial, pulse 104/min (regular), BP 110/60 mmHg. Heart sounds are normal. Chest examination reveals a few scattered wheezes. Neurological examination is normal. ECG shows sinus tachycardia with inverted T waves in leads V1-V3. Chest radiography normal. Oxygen saturation is 92% on 40% oxygen. PEFR is 290 L/min. What is the most likely diagnosis?

A acute pulmonary oedema

B acute exacerbation of chronic obstructive pulmonary disease

C pulmonary embolism

D acute myocardial infarction

E pneumocystis

Respiratory medicine

Praveen Bhatia, Michael I Polkey *(Editor)*
and Veronica LC White

Respiratory Medicine

Answers are on pp. 132–134.

Question 143

A 45-year-old man who smoked 15 cigarettes/day for 20 years, but stopped 3 years ago, now presents with cough and malaise. He had a deep venous thrombosis of his right leg 20 years previously after an operation to remove a cartilage from his right knee, but otherwise he has no significant past medical history, takes no regular medications, and physical examination is normal. His chest radiograph is shown (Figure 20). The most likely diagnosis is:

A lung cancer
B sarcoidosis
C pulmonary hypertension
D pneumonia
E interstitial lung disease

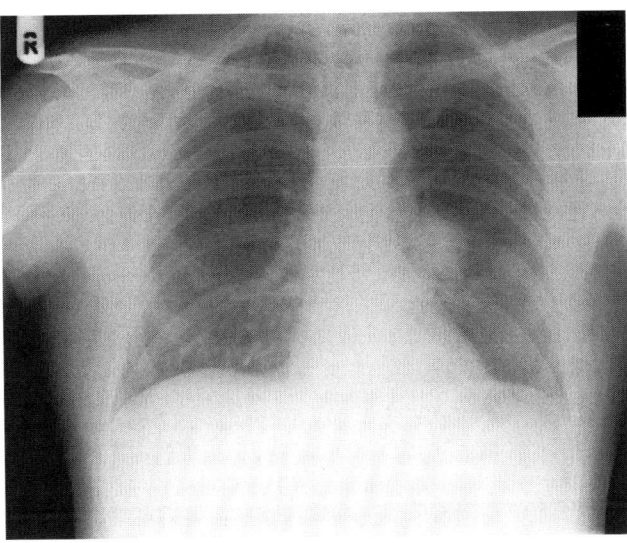

Fig. 20 Question 143.

Question 144

A 62-year-old man who smoked 10 cigarettes/day for 15 years, but stopped smoking about 30 years ago, presents with a month's history of breathlessness. He assumed that this was due to a 'chest infection', but matters have not improved, leading him to seek medical attention. He may have had a 'bit of a temperature', but he has had no other respiratory symptoms and physical examination is normal. His chest radiograph is shown (Figure 21). The diagnosis is:

A left lower lobe collapse
B right middle lobe collapse
C right upper lobe collapse
D left pneumothorax
E chronic obstructive pulmonary disease

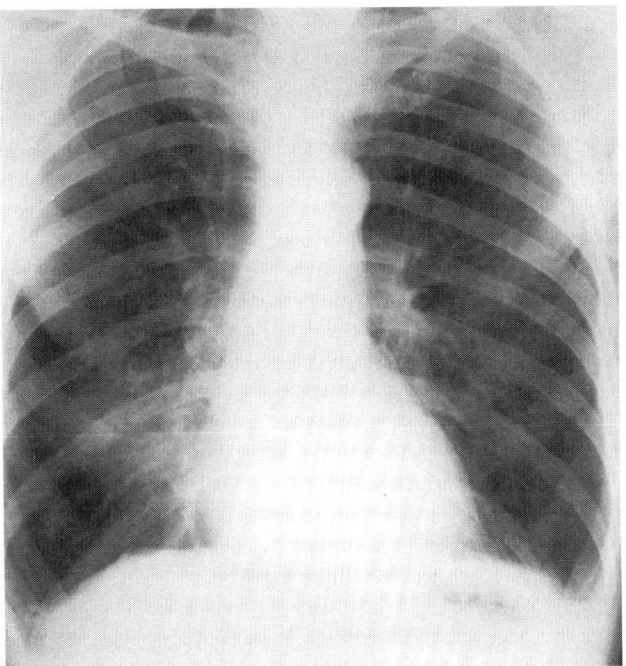

Fig. 21 Question 144.

Question 145

A 35-year-old postman presents with a history of breathlessness that has been getting gradually worse over 6 months. He coughs up sputum regularly, but is otherwise well, with no significant past medical history. He smoked five to ten cigarettes per day from the age of 18 to 26 years. The two most likely diagnoses are:

A cystic fibrosis
B emphysema
C congestive cardiac failure
D alpha-1 antitrypsin deficiency

E pneumoconiosis

F asbestosis

G hypogammaglobulinaemia

H chronic obstructive pulmonary disease

I bronchial asthma

J postman's lung

Question 146

A 38-year-old woman presents with a two-year history of worsening breathlessness. Results of preliminary investigation are as follows: spirometry – Forced Expiratory Volume in one second (FEV1) 83% predicted, Vital Capacity (VC) 79% predicted, FEV1/VC ratio 78%; chest radiograph reported as being within normal limits; blood gases (breathing air) – PaO_2 9.6 kPa, $PaCO_2$ 4.1 kPa. What are the two most likely diagnoses?

A chronic obstructive pulmonary disease

B cardiac failure

C diffuse parenchymal lung disease

D pneumocystis carinii pneumonia

E anaemia

F bronchiectasis

G asthma

H pulmonary vascular disease

I diabetes mellitus

J primary hyperventilation

Question 147

A 36-year-old woman is admitted with a history of cough and shortness of breath of 8 weeks' duration. Her chest radiograph shows bilateral mid-zone infiltrates and blood count shows a raised eosinophil count. Which two of the following drugs might be responsible for her condition?

A bleomycin

B amiodarone

C calcium tablets

D prednisolone

E heroin

F insulin

G cyclophosphamide

H busulfan

I sulfasalazine

J paracetamol

Question 148

A 56-year-old woman, a smoker of 20 cigarettes daily, presents with a 6-month history of progressive shortness of breath. Her past medical history is unremarkable apart from Raynaud's syndrome for which she takes a calcium channel blocker. On examination no significant abnormality is found apart from telangiectasia. Her chest radiograph shows clear lung fields, prominent pulmonary arteries and mildly enlarged heart. Spirometry is normal, but gas transfer is reduced to 50% predicted. What is the most likely diagnosis?

A cor pulmonale secondary to chronic obstructive pulmonary disease

B multiple pulmonary emboli

C pulmonary arterial hypertension

D sarcoidosis

E congestive cardiac failure

Question 149

A 63-year-old man attends the hospital with a history of proximal muscle weakness. He also gives a history of a cough of 8 weeks duration and complains of pain in the small joints of the hands. On examination he has small haemorrhages in the nail folds, but is not clubbed. There are bi-basal crackles, and a chest radiograph reveals diffuse reticular infiltrates. Lung function tests confirm a restrictive pattern. What is the underlying cause of his interstitial lung disease?

A cryptogenic fibrosing alveolitis

B ankylosing spondylitis

C polymyositis/dermatomyositis

D rheumatoid arthritis

E mixed connective tissue disorder

Question 150

A 26-year-old man is admitted with a history of 4–6 weeks of breathlessness. He initially had 'flu-like symptoms and was treated by his doctor with a 10-day course of ciprofloxacin. However, he then started coughing up blood, leading to urgent referral. On examination he is breathless at rest, with bilateral crackles in the lungs. Investigation reveals anaemia and impaired renal function (creatinine 220 µmol/l). Pulmonary function tests are normal apart from an abnormally high transfer factor. Urine dipstick testing shows the presence of red blood cells. What is the most likely diagnosis?

A pneumococcal pneumonia with post-streptococcal nephritis

B Goodpasture's syndrome

C chronic eosinophilic pneumonia

D bronchiolitis obliterans

E Churg-Strauss

Question 151

A 35-year-old woman is referred with a history of red, painful legs of 3 weeks duration that have not responded to a course of amoxycillin and flucloxacillin given for presumed cellulitis. She is afebrile, does not have any other symptoms, and has never smoked. Examination reveals tender purple/red nodules on her shins. Her full blood count, kidney and liver function tests are normal. A chest radiograph shows prominent hilae. What is the appropriate management?

A arrange bronchoscopy and bronchoalveolar lavage to exclude malignancy

B start azathioprine and prednisolone; follow up in clinic

C start prednisolone; follow up in clinic

D start simple analgesics; follow up in clinic

E arrange CT scan of the lungs and lung biopsy

Question 152

A 65-year-old woman is admitted with left sided pneumonia and pleural effusion. Pleural fluid is aspirated and sent for testing. Which of the following is an indication for inserting a chest drain?

A pleural fluid pH < 7.2

B serous pleural fluid

C blood stained pleural fluid

D pleural fluid glucose >2 mmol/l

E pleural fluid lactate dehydrogenase >200 IU/l

Question 153

A 78-year-old man is referred to the chest clinic with history of dyspnoea for over 3 months. He is a retired teacher and has never smoked. He has a past medical history of atrial fibrillation, which is well controlled on digoxin. He also takes warfarin and the occasional paracetamol. He is clubbed and hypoxic on air with a SaO_2 of 89%. He has bilateral crackles and a chest radiograph confirms fibrosing alveolitis. Which of the following combination of lung function is typical of this condition?

A reduced FEV1 & FVC, FEV1/FVC < 70%, raised TLC & RV, reduced TLCO

B reduced FEV1 & FVC, FEV1/FVC > 70%, raised TLC & RV, reduced TLCO

C normal FEV1 & FVC, FEV1/FVC > 70%, raised TLC & RV, reduced TLCO

D reduced FEV1 & FVC, FEV1/FVC > 70%, reduced TLC & RV, reduced TLCO

E reduced FEV1 & FVC, FEV1/FVC > 70%, raised TLC & RV, normal TLCO

Question 154

A 40-year-old man, a smoker of 40 pack years, presents with a 3-month history of shortness of breath. His past medical history includes hypertension, cervical spondylosis and depression. Spirometry shows Forced Expiratory Volume in one second (FEV1) of 1.03 litres – 67% predicted, Forced Vital Capacity (FVC) 1.03 litres – 53% predicted, and FEV1/FVC of 96%. How would you interpret his spirometry results?

A normal for his age

B obstructive defect

C mixed defect

D restrictive defect

E unable to interpret as bronchial reversibility not done

Question 155

A 43-year-old woman presents with breathlessness that has been getting gradually worse over a few weeks and now makes it difficult for her to walk upstairs. On physical examination she is found to have a large left sided pleural effusion but no other abnormalities. The presence of the effusion is confirmed by chest radiography. The most appropriate initial investigation would be:

A CT chest

B diagnostic aspiration of pleural fluid followed by drainage of effusion to dryness

C diagnostic aspiration of pleural fluid with pleural biopsy

D sputum cytology

E diagnostic aspiration of pleural fluid

Question 156

A 65-year-old man presents with a history of worsening breathlessness and cough. His arterial blood gases (breathing air) show the following: pH 7.26, pO_2 6.5 kPa, pCO_2 9.5 kPa, bicarbonate 32 mmol/L. Which of the following is the most likely diagnosis?

A obstructive sleep apnoea

B acute asthma

C pulmonary embolism

D acute exacerbation of chronic obstructive pulmonary disease

E pulmonary oedema

Question 157

You are called to the resuscitation room to see a 25-year-old man whose condition has suddenly deteriorated. He had arrived 30 minutes earlier with a 2-hour history of central pleuritic chest pain and breathlessness. He collapsed while awaiting a chest radiograph and now is agitated and cyanosed with pulse 120/min and BP 80/40 mmHg. Oxygen saturation is reading 79%, with the patient breathing high flow oxygen via a re-breathe mask. Respiratory examination reveals reduced breath sounds in the right lung field with deviation of the trachea towards the left. Percussion is resonant bilaterally. What immediate course of action should you take?

A arrange for urgent portable chest radiograph
B contact the Intensive Care Unit to arrange for the patient to be ventilated
C insert large bore needle into left hemithorax
D insert large bore needle into right hemithorax
E check arterial blood gases and commence BiPAP if hypoxia is confirmed

Gastroenterology and hepatology

Jane D Collier *(Editor)*, John M Hebden,
Satish Keshav and Jeremy Shearman

Gastroenterology and Hepatology

Answers are on pp. 134–137.

Question 158

A 58-year-old woman with autosomal dominant poly-cystic kidney disease presents with increasing abdominal discomfort and distention. A CT scan of her abdomen is shown (see Figure 22). What does this show?

A polycystic kidneys

B polycystic kidneys and polycystic liver

C polycystic kidneys, polycystic liver and ascites

D polycystic kidneys and ascites

E polycystic liver and ascites

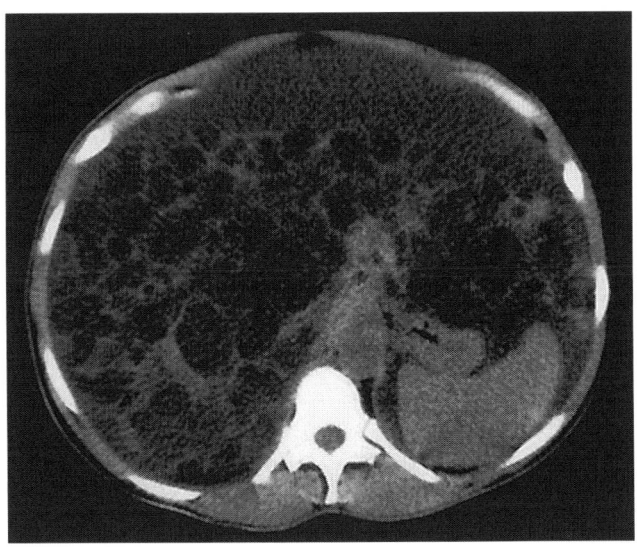

Fig. 22 Question 158.

Question 159

A 68-year-old man with a past history of severe sero-positive rheumatoid arthritis presents with difficulty swallowing, such that on a couple of occasions he has 'almost choked' after eating bread. He has lost about a stone in weight over the last couple of months. On examination he has musculoskeletal deformities due to his rheumatoid arthritis and he looks unwell and a bit pale, but there are no other abnormalities. His barium swallow is shown (see Figure 23). What is the likely diagnosis?

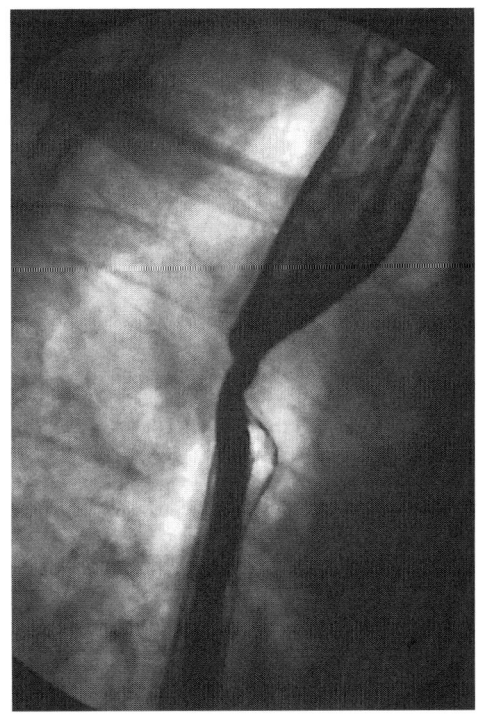

Fig. 23 Question 159.

A achalasia

B malignant oesophageal stricture

C benign oesophageal stricture

D hiatus hernia

E post-cricoid web

Question 160

A 47-year-old man presents with a 1 day history of increasing confusion, drowsiness and jaundice. He has been suffering from depression for the last 6 months, but has no other significant past medical history. The two most likely causes of his acute liver failure are:

A hepatitis A

B autoimmune chronic active hepatitis

C primary biliary cirrhosis

D hepatitis B

E Budd Chiari syndrome

F paracetamol overdose

G hepatitis C

H leptospirosis

I drug induced (not paracetamol)

J Wilson's disease

Question 161

A 35-year-old white English woman presents with abdominal pain and vomiting. She has been unwell for about six weeks with anorexia, nausea and weight loss. Examination reveals a tender palpable mass in the right iliac fossa. The two most likely diagnoses are:

A psoas abscess

B tuberculosis

C abdominal secondaries

D Crohn's disease

E *Campylobacter*

F caecal carcinoma

G hypernephroma

H appendix mass

I ovarian carcinoma

J lymphoma

Question 162

You are called to review a 67-year-old man admitted 4 days ago with central abdominal pain. A diagnosis of acute pancreatitis was made clinically and biochemically, and the surgeons have managed him conservatively. A few small gallbladder stones were noted on ultrasonography, but the common bile duct was not dilated and no stones were seen in the duct. A CT scan has been requested. He is a strict Muslim whose only other past medical history is ulcerative colitis, for which he is on treatment with prednisolone and azathioprine. The two most likely causes of his pancreatitis are:

A alcohol-induced

B hereditary

C drug-induced

D gallstones

E idiopathic

F hyperparathyroidism

G mumps infection

H pancreas divisum

I trauma

J CMV infection

Question 163

A 35-year-old woman, otherwise fit and well, presents with isolated transaminitis. She denies excess alcohol use and ultrasound of her liver reveals only fatty change. Her standard liver screen is negative. Which statement best reflects this clinical scenario?

A she most likely has non A-E hepatitis and should be screened for hepatitis G

B silent alcohol abuse should be assumed

C non-alcoholic fatty liver disease is most likely

D Wilson's disease needs to be excluded by liver biopsy

E she should be advised that she cannot be a blood donor

Question 164

A 43-year-old man presents with an acute colitic illness and is passing between five and ten bloody stools per day. Which one of the following statements is true?

A steroids are contraindicated until negative stool culture results have been obtained

B approximately 30% of cases of acute severe ulcerative colitis (UC) occur in newly diagnosed cases

C *Clostridium difficile* always produces characteristic endoscopic and histological changes

D the finding of cytomegalovirus (CMV) inclusion bodies in biopsy samples is conclusive evidence for a pathogenic role and mandates intravenous ganciclovir instead of intravenous corticosteroid

E amoebic dysentery can be safely discounted as a possible cause five years after last travel in the tropics

Question 165

An 83-year-old man is about to be discharged home, having spent 3 weeks in hospital being treated for *C. difficile* diarrhoea associated with pseudomembranous colitis. Unfortunately, the nursing staff report that he has had a recurrence of profuse, malodorous, greenish diarrhoea. He has already had one course of oral metronidazole therapy. Which of the following is the most appropriate treatment?

A intravenous metronidazole

B oral metronidazole

C intravenous teicoplanin

D intravenous vancomycin

E oral ciprofloxacin

Question 166

A 21-year-old student develops abdominal pain, fever and diarrhoea 12 hours after eating a chicken sandwich that had been in his fridge for a week. The most likely cause is:

A *Campylobacter*
B Norwalk virus
C *Salmonella*
D *E. coli* O157
E *Giardia*

Question 167

A 30-year-old woman with long standing medically treated Crohn's disease presents to clinic with increasing abdominal pain associated with intermittent vomiting and bloating. Her inflammatory markers are normal. Which is the most likely cause of her symptoms?

A exacerbation of colonic colitis
B stricture formation secondary to long standing disease
C colovesical fistula
D adhesions
E colorectal cancer

Question 168

A 70-year-old woman presents with watery diarrhoea. Flexible sigmoidoscopy is reported as normal but histology shows a lymphocytic infiltration. Which of the following best describes optimum management and complications?

A the patient should be warned about an increased risk of colorectal carcinoma
B non-steroidal anti-inflammatory drugs (NSAIDs) are unlikely to have caused her symptoms and can safely be continued
C toxic megacolon is a common complication
D budesonide is effective treatment
E collagenous colitis has a similar microscopic appearance

Question 169

A previously fit 35-year-old man presents with pyrexia and tachycardia, severe bloody diarrhoea and mucus per rectum. His symptoms have been present for three weeks. The most likely diagnosis is:

A ischaemic colitis
B bacterial colitis
C ulcerative colitis
D protozoal colitis
E non-steroidal anti-inflammatory drug (NSAID) induced colitis

Question 170

A 35-year-old woman presents with abdominal bloating, change in the form of her stool with nocturnal diarrhoea, abdominal pain relieved by defaecation, and marked gastrocolic reflex. Which one of these features is NOT a feature of Irritable Bowel Syndrome:

A bloating
B change in the form of the stool
C nocturnal diarrhoea
D abdominal pain relieved with defaecation
E marked gastrocolic reflex

Question 171

A 60-year-old man with known ulcerative colitis and diverticular disease comes to clinic complaining of passing faeces per urethra. Cystoscopy confirms a fistula between his bladder and bowel. Which treatment is most likely to be effective?

A total parenteral nutrition (TPN)
B steroids
C antibiotics
D surgery
E elemental diet

Question 172

A 70-year-old man presents to casualty with lower abdominal pain and fever. He is not jaundiced and blood analysis reveals only a raised white cell count, with normal liver function tests. Previous upper GI endoscopy is reported as normal and urinalysis and MSU are normal. What is the most likely diagnosis?

A cholecystitis
B diverticulitis
C gastritis
D carcinoma of the bowel
E pyelonephritis

Question 173

You are asked to review a 45-year-old man recovering from a road traffic accident, just off intensive care. Although able to eat and drink small amounts he remains generally weak and has lost 20% of his pre-morbid weight. His bowels are working normally. The orthopaedic team ask your advice regarding his nutrition. What do you recommend?

A regular monitoring of his weight, only taking action if he fails to put weight on in the next 7 days
B insertion of a tunnelled central venous line for parenteral nutrition
C booking him for percutaneous endoscopic gastrostomy (PEG) at the earliest available opportunity
D oral dietary supplements

E insertion of a naso-gastric tube and commencement of supplemental enteral nutrition as soon as possible

Question 174

A 28-year-old man complains of a 3-year history of difficulty swallowing both solids and liquids. A barium meal shows a slightly dilated oesophagus and subsequent endoscopy is normal apart from oesophageal candidiasis. The next best investigation is:

A anti-Ro and anti-La antibodies
B fasting glucose
C oesophageal manometry
D CT thorax
E the edrophonium chloride (Tensilon) test

Question 175

A 65-year-old man complains of epigastric pain and difficulty swallowing. At endoscopy Grade I reflux oesophagitis is seen. Which one of the following statements is NOT true?

A acid suppression with a proton pump inhibitor should relieve symptoms
B repeat endoscopy is required to ascertain response to treatment
C *Helicobacter* eradication is not needed unless there is associated duodenitis
D raising the head of the bed and avoiding eating/drinking 3 hours prior to going to bed can aid symptoms.
E the lowest dose of proton pump inhibitor should be used in the long term to treat his symptoms.

Question 176

A 70-year-old man with dysphagia is seen in clinic. He is unable to swallow any solids or fluids. What is the best course of action?

A admit the patient from clinic for further investigations
B arrange a CT abdomen and chest to look for metastatic cancer
C arrange an appointment in the combined oncology-surgery clinic
D prescribe high dose proton pump inhibitors (PPIs) to reduce acid reflux
E book the patient for percutaneous endoscopic gastrostomy (PEG) insertion

Question 177

A 78-year-old woman is admitted on take because she is unable to cope at home. She says that she feels 'a bit weak'

but admits to no other symptoms. On examination she looks as though she has lost a lot of weight and is jaundiced, but there are no other abnormal physical signs. The most likely diagnosis is:

A gall stones
B carcinoma of the stomach with hilar lymph nodes
C chronic pancreatitis
D carcinoma of the pancreas
E cholangiocarcinoma

Question 178

A 55-year-old man is still anaemic, has some loose stools and has failed to regain weight several months after starting a gluten-free diet for coeliac disease. Which of the following is the commonest cause of failure to respond to treatment?

A pancreatic insufficiency
B dietary non-compliance
C small bowel adenocarcinoma
D enteropathy associated B cell lymphoma of the small intestine
E ulcerative jejunitis

Question 179

A 68-year-old woman presents with a six-month history of diarrhoea and weight loss. Extensive investigation eventually culminates in the finding of multiple diverticula on a small bowel enema. The first-line treatment should be:

A augmentin for 10 days
B laparotomy and resection of the affected bowel
C metronidazole for 10 days
D vancomycin for 10 days
E trial of lactose-free diet

Question 180

A 30-year-old woman is seen with weight loss and diarrhoea. Three years ago she spent 6 months in Egypt. Previous investigations have included negative endomysial antibodies, normal hydrogen breath test and normal barium follow through. Which method is the most appropriate way of diagnosing chronic giardiasis?

A urine culture
B serology
C histology from the second part of the duodenum
D colonoscopic appearances
E small bowel enteroscopy

Question 181

A 46-year-old man presents with jaundice. Dipstick testing of his urine reveals the presence of bilirubin but no urobilinogen. This means that:

A jaundice is likely to be pre-hepatic

B bile must be flowing freely into the gut

C jaundice cannot be obstructive

D renal function is normal

E there must be complete obstruction to bile flow

Question 182

A 58-year-old man presents with diarrhoea and weight loss. Amongst many investigations he has a lactulose breath test. The reason for the test is to detect:

A diarrhoea due to laxative consumption

B bacterial overgrowth in the small bowel

C hypolactasia

D infection with *H pylori*

E malabsorption due to small intestinal disease

Neurology

Gillian L Hall, Aroon D Hingorani,
John P Patten, Sivakumar Sathasivam
and Nick Ward *(Editor)*

Neurology

Answers are on pp. 137–140.

Question 183

A 48-year-old man presents with unsteadiness of gait and double-vision. Figure 24 shows the appearance of his eyes when he attempts to look to his left. What is the diagnosis?

A left third nerve palsy

B left fourth nerve palsy

C left sixth nerve palsy

D right third nerve palsy

E right third nerve palsy

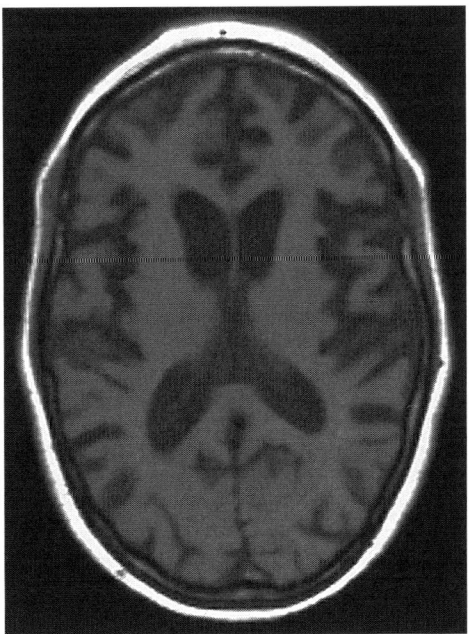

Fig. 25 Question 184.

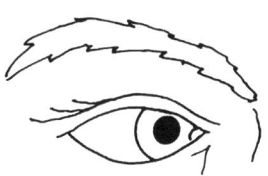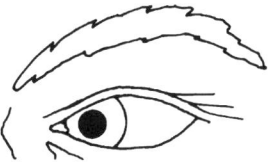

Fig. 24 Question 183.

Question 184

A 78-year-old woman presents on the general medical take with falls, cognitive impairment and failure to cope at home. Her abbreviated mental test score is 2/10 and her gait is very unsteady. A CT scan of her brain is done (see Figure 25). What is the diagnosis?

A bilateral subdural haemorrhages

B normal pressure hydrocephalus

C obstructive hydrocephalus

D cerebral atrophy

E multi-infarct picture

Question 185

A 58-year-old man presents complaining of unsteadiness. Which two of the following symptoms or signs would usually be inconsistent with a cerebellar lesion?

A symptoms worse in dark

B symptoms have got worse over several years

C symptoms are very brief and associated with head movement

D sustained horizontal nystagmus that does not fatigue

E a wide-based gait

F bilateral upgoing plantars

G papilloedema

H headache

I diplopia

J pain in the neck and wasting of hand muscles.

Question 186

A 68-year-old woman is referred having had a 'funny turn', the question asked by the general practitioner being 'was this a transient ischaemic attack (TIA)?' Which two features listed below would be acceptable to sustain the diagnosis of TIA?

A vertigo

B diplopia

C dysphagia

D dysphasia

E dysphonia

F loss of balance

75

G tinnitus
H impairment of the function of one hand
I amnesia
J sensory symptoms confined to one part of limb or face

Question 187

A 16-year-old girl presents with a history of episodes of bizarre behaviour following her parents' recent divorce. Her mother describes these attacks to you. Which two of the following features would suggest a true epileptic seizure rather than a non-epileptic attack?

A limb flailing
B opisthotonus
C carpet burns
D tongue biting
E pelvic thrusting
F duration of several hours
G cyanosis
H rapid recovery
I directed violent behaviour
J repetitive chewing movements

Question 188

A 40-year-old man presents with progressive leg weakness. Which two features would be AGAINST a diagnosis of Guillain-Barré syndrome?

A severe back pain
B recent chest infection
C urinary incontinence at the beginning of the illness
D fluctuating blood pressure
E sluggish pupillary reactions
F normal arm and leg reflexes
G marked fatigability of leg movement
H subjective sensory disturbance
I dysarthria
J shortness of breath on exertion

Question 189

A 19-year-old man presents with a history of a single tonic-clonic seizure that occurred the morning after a party. On direct questioning he also reports the occurrence of occasional blank spells and brief jerking of his upper limbs several times a month. Which of the following drugs is most suitable?

A phenytoin
B carbamazepine
C sodium valproate

D gabapentin
E clonazepam

Question 190

A 30-year-old man presents with a tremor. He has had this for many years, but it has become worse recently such that he now finds it socially embarrassing. His father had a similar problem. His gait is normal. The most likely diagnosis is:

A Wilson's disease
B familial cerebellar degeneration
C Parkinson's disease
D Huntington's disease
E benign essential tremor

Question 191

An 82-year-old man is admitted following a fall. The physiotherapist thinks he looks Parkinsonian and asks for your opinion. Which of the following is most supportive of a diagnosis of Parkinson's disease?

A his tremor is most disabling when he is drinking his tea
B his neck is extended and he has a surprised expression, despite paucity of facial movement
C the tremor is worse in his left arm and leg
D you elicit a positive glabellar tap
E you notice marked oro-facial dyskinesia

Question 192

A 29-year-old man presents with a 9-month history of depression, 4-month history of painful sensory disturbance in both legs, and most recently cognitive impairment with myoclonus. His MRI scan reveals thalamic hyperintensity on T2-weighted images. His EEG is normal. The most likely diagnosis is:

A corticobasal degeneration
B progressive multifocal leucoencephalopathy
C juvenile myoclonic epilepsy
D new variant Creutzfeldt-Jakob disease
E Wilson's disease

Question 193

A patient presents with high stepping gait. Which of the following is the most likely diagnosis?

A cerebellar lesion
B diffuse cerebrovascular disease
C Parkinson's disease
D peripheral neuropathy
E proximal myopathy

Question 194

A 65-year-old man presents with a 3-month history of dysarthria and progressive difficulty in swallowing. Examination reveals a weak, fasciculating, spastic tongue and a brisk gag reflex and jaw jerk. The likely diagnosis is:

A basilar artery thrombosis

B multiple sclerosis

C Miller–Fisher syndrome

D amyotrophic lateral sclerosis

E Wernicke's encephalopathy

Question 195

A 56-year-old woman presents with progressive leg weakness over 3 days. She has noted minor urinary incontinence in addition. She has a past medical history of breast cancer treated 10 year ago with lumpectomy and radiotherapy. Which is the investigation of choice?

A myelography

B plain spinal radiographs

C lumbar puncture

D computed tomography (CT)

E magnetic resonance imaging (MRI)

Question 196

A patient presents with weakness of knee extension and ankle inversion. Which of the following nerve roots is most likely affected?

A L2

B L3

C L4

D L5

E S1

Question 197

A 65-year-old man presents with pain and weakness in his left arm. Which one of the following features is NOT consistent with a C5/C6 radiculopathy?

A weakness of deltoid muscle

B reduced biceps reflex

C sensory loss over the ring and little finger

D weakness of supraspinatus muscle

E winging of the scapula

Question 198

A 30-year-old man describes recurrent daily attacks of severe constant unilateral orbital pain over the last 2 months. He tends to get bouts of this type of attack once to twice a year, typically lasting six to eight weeks in duration. Which of the following would be appropriate prophylactic treatment?

A amitriptyline

B carbamazepine

C pizotifen

D propranolol

E verapamil

Question 199

A 43-year-old man complains of sensory loss in his left arm and hand. On examination he has subjectively diminished light touch and pinprick sensation in the left hand extending to above the elbow. Joint position sense appears intact. With his eyes closed, he has difficulty distinguishing his cigarette lighter from a pen using the left hand, and his two-point discrimination is 11 mm. Which investigation is most likely to be diagnostic?

A CT head

B electromyogram (EMG) and nerve conduction studies

C MRI cervical spine

D chest radiograph

E vitamin B12 levels

Question 200

A 36-year-old man presents with a few days of low back pain that radiates to his buttocks and is associated with lower limb parathesiae. He now has difficulty walking, particularly on uneven surfaces. The reflexes are difficult to elicit. The most likely cause is:

A acute lumbar disc prolapse

B vertebral collapse secondary to malignant infiltration

C acute porphyria

D Guillain–Barré syndrome

E post infectious transverse myelitis

Question 201

A 58-year-old man presents with back pain that radiates through the knee and down the medial side of the calf to the medial malleolus. The nerve root involved is:

A L2

B L3

C L4

D L5

E S1

Question 202

You are examining the pupils of a 48-year-old woman in whom the diagnosis of multiple sclerosis is suspected. Which of the following observations would make you conclude that she has a left relative afferent pupillary defect?

A you move a light from her left eye to her right eye, and the left pupil constricts

B you move a light from her right eye to her left eye, and the left pupil dilates

C you flash a light on and off in her right eye, and the left pupil constricts, but it does not when you flash it on and off in her left eye

D you move a light from her right eye to her left eye, and the left pupil constricts

E you move a light from her left eye to her right eye, and the left pupil dilates

Question 203

A 38-year-old woman has weakness of her right foot. You are trying to decide whether she has a common peroneal nerve lesion or an L5 root lesion. Which of the following statements is true?

A an L5 root lesion will cause sensory and motor symptoms, but a common peroneal nerve lesion will only cause motor symptoms

B a common peroneal nerve lesion will cause weakness of ankle dorsiflexion, eversion and inversion, but an L5 root lesion will not affect inversion

C an L5 root lesion will cause loss of the ankle jerk, but a common peroneal nerve lesion will not

D a common peroneal nerve lesion will cause weakness of ankle dorsiflexion and eversion but will not affect inversion, which will be affected in an L5 root lesion

E the two conditions cannot be distinguished clinically, but can by nerve conduction studies

Ophthalmology

Peggy Frith *(Editor)* and Hamish MA Towler

Ophthalmology

Answers are on p. 140.

Question 204

A 38-year-old woman presents with blurring of vision in her right eye that has developed over the last 3 days. She says that she can now see very little out of it, and acuity is reduced to counting fingers. The optic fundus is shown (see Figure 26). What is the diagnosis?

A papilloedema

B optic neuritis

C central retinal artery occlusion

D central retinal vein occlusion

E optic atrophy

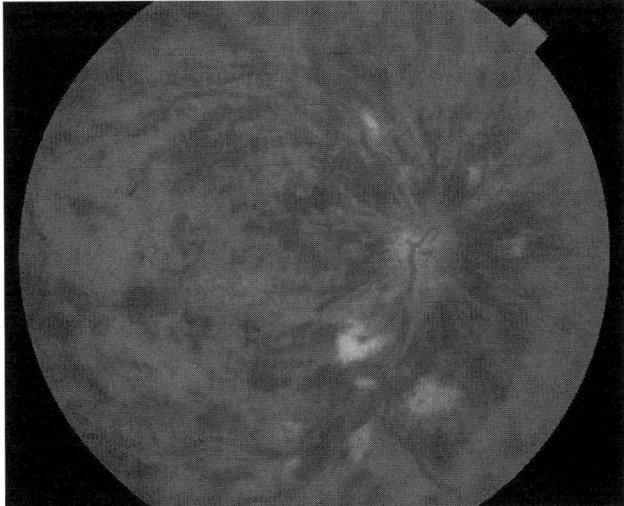

Fig. 27 Question 205.

D vitreous haemorrhage

E acute glaucoma

Question 206

A 48-year-old man with diabetes finds that the vision in one eye is blurred when he reads, but not at other times. The most likely diagnosis is:

A macular oedema

B floaters

C cataract

D glaucoma

E stroke

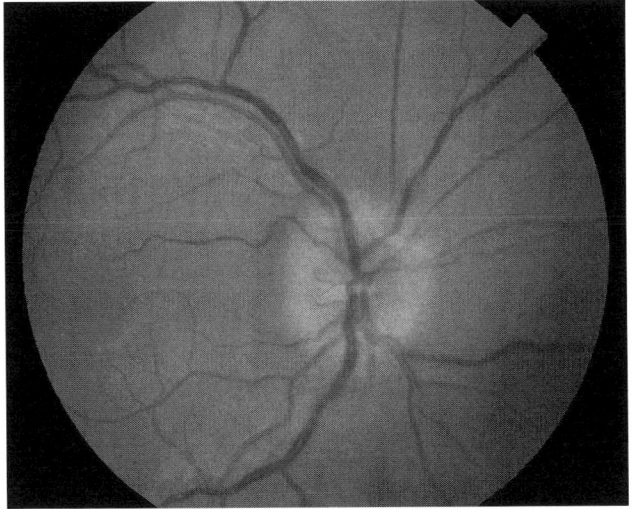

Fig. 26 Question 204.

Question 205

A 60-year-old man with type 2 diabetes mellitus reported that when watching television 'something went wrong with his vision'. The optic fundus of his right eye is shown (see Figure 27). What is the diagnosis?

A papilloedema with fundal haemorrhages and exudates

B central retinal artery occlusion

C central retinal vein occlusion

Question 207

A 50-year-old diabetic woman with ischaemic heart disease complains of a problem with the vision in her left eye. To get a good view of the ocular fundi for diagnostic purposes the best agent to dilate her pupils with is:

A cyclopentolate 1%

B tropicamide 0.5%

C tropicamide 1%

D phenylephrine 2.5%

E phenylephrine 10%

Psychiatry

**Vincent Kirchner and
Maurice Lipsedge** *(Editor)*

Psychiatry

Answers are on pp. 140–141.

Question 208

A 40-year-old man from Uganda is brought in by the police under section 136 of the Mental Health Act. He was arrested because he was standing naked in a busy street attempting to 'direct' the traffic. On examination he declared that he was the Minister of Transport. He spoke rapidly and paced around the room issuing orders in a loud voice. He was found to have oral thrush. From the following choose the two LEAST likely diagnostic possibilities:

A mania

B tertiary Syphilis

C amphetamine use

D gonorrhoea

E adverse effects of antiretroviral drugs

F neuropsychiatric sequelae of HIV

G delirium due to secondary infection

H cocaine use

I post traumatic stress disorder

J psychological reaction to the diagnosis of AIDS

Question 209

A very thin 18-year-old girl is referred for investigation of weight loss. You suspect that she has anorexia nervosa, but perform a range of screening tests. Which one of the following would be compatible with the diagnosis of anorexia nervosa?

A hyperkalaemia

B low serum bicarbonate

C low serum cholesterol

D low white cell count

E elevated ESR

Question 210

A 78-year-old man, without significant past medical history and taking no regular medications, has become increasingly forgetful over the last 18 months, to the point where he now finds it difficult to remember the names of some members of his family. He has recently been having visual hallucinations. On examination he seems rather expressionless and has cogwheel rigidity of both arms. The most likely diagnosis is:

A Alzheimer's disease

B Lewy body dementia

C vascular dementia

D frontal lobe dementia

E Alzheimer's disease and Parkinson's disease.

Question 211

A 42-year-old woman is referred to the medical out-patient clinic because she is 'always exhausted'. She says that she cannot do anything that requires any physical effort and that she sleeps all the time. Her general practitioner cannot find any explanation for her symptoms. You consider the diagnosis of chronic fatigue syndrome. Which one of the following findings would NOT be consistent with this diagnosis?

A subjective memory impairment

B tender lymph nodes

C muscle pain

D joint pain

E weight loss

Endocrinology

Anna Crown, Paul D Flynn,
Mark Gurnell *(Editor)* and
Mohammed Z Qureshi

Endocrinology

Answers are on pp. 141–145.

Question 212

A 48-year-old woman with known Graves' disease, presents with double vision that is worst when she tries to look to her left side. Figure 28 shows her trying to do this: what does it reveal?

A proptosis of right eye

B bilateral lid retraction and left sixth nerve palsy

C bilateral lid retraction and lid lag of right eye

D bilateral lid retraction and proptosis of right eye

E lid lag of right eye

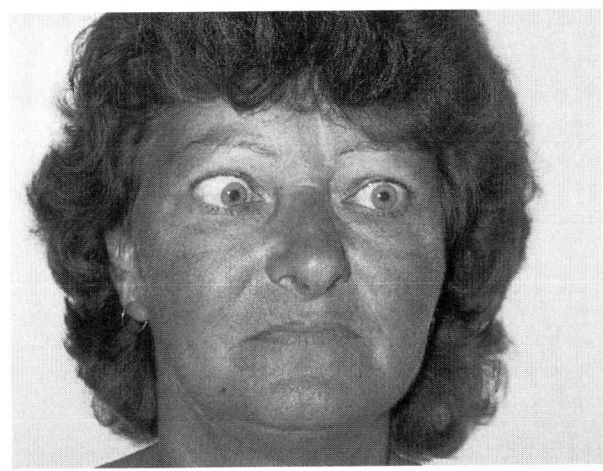

Fig. 28 Question 212.

Question 213

A 53-year-old man presents with impotence that has been troubling him for some years. He is otherwise well. Figure 29 shows his face. What is the likely diagnosis?

A hypogonadism

B hypothyroidism

C hypoadrenalism (Addison's disease)

D amyloidosis

E acromegaly

Question 214

A 78-year-old woman presents 'off legs' on the general medical take. She appears very frail and malnourished and

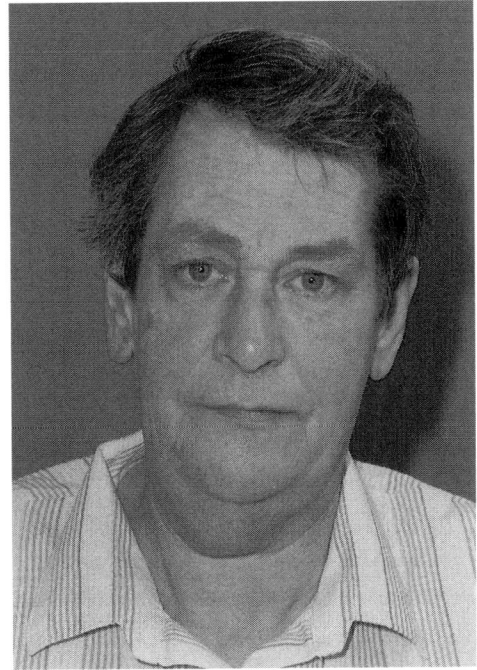

Fig. 29 Question 213.

clearly in pain from her hips and / or pelvis when she tries to get up and walk. Figure 30 shows a radiograph of her pelvis, hips and proximal femurs. What is the likely diagnosis?

A osteomalacia

B osteoporosis

C myeloma

D polymyalgia rheumatica

E Paget's disease

Question 215

Which two of the following would NOT be on your list of differential diagnoses for the cause of a corrected serum calcium level of 3.2 mmol/l in a 61-year-old woman?

A tuberculosis

B osteoporosis

C berylliosis

D Addison's disease

E Paget's disease

F primary hyperparathyroidism

G secondary hyperparathyroidism

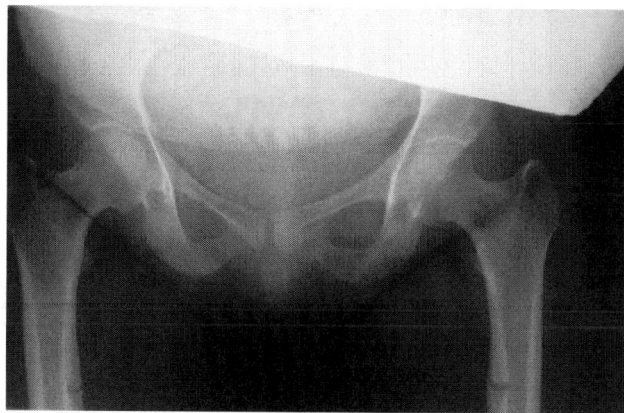

Fig. 30 Question 214.

H tertiary hyperparathyroidism

I bendrofluazide medication

J lithium medication

Question 216

A 60-year-old woman of Gujrati origin presents with a 6-month history of generalised aches and pains. Her corrected calcium is 1.67 mmol/l with albumin of 38 g/l. Her creatinine is 88 μmol/l, alkaline phosphatse 560 U/l, phosphate 0.80 mmol/l and parathyroid hormone (PTH) level is 173 pg/ml (upper limit of normal: 80 pg/ml). Which two of the following conditions does she have?

A primary hyperparathyroidism

B osteoporosis

C pseudopseudohypoparathyroidism

D previous thyroidectomy

E ectopic PTH production

F chronic renal failure

G secondary hyperparathyroidism

H Paget's disease

I tertiary hyperparathyroidism

J osteomalacia

Question 217

A 33-year-old man is referred to the endocrine clinic for routine follow-up having recently moved into the region. He has previously undergone a total parathyroidectomy for hyperparathyroidism arising in the setting of multiple endocrine neoplasia type 1 (MEN1), a diagnosis that has been confirmed by genetic screening. Even in the absence of symptoms, it would be appropriate to check which two of the following biochemical parameters?

A fasting calcitonin

B serum prolactin

C urinary catecholamines

D urinary 5 hydroxyindoleacetic acid (5-HIAA)

E serum corrected calcium

F free T3

G serum ferritin

H cortisol response to synacthen

I plasma glucose

J serum thyroid stimulating hormone (TSH)

Question 218

A 59-year-old man is referred with weight loss, sweating and palpitation of three months' duration. He denies any other symptoms and his past history is notable only for a myocardial infarction 3 years previously with subsequent episodes of ventricular tachycardia. His medication consists of aspirin 75 mg od, pravastatin 40 mg on, ramipril 10 mg od, atenolol 50 mg od and amiodarone 200 mg od. Which two of the following are true?

A free thyroxine would be the most informative test

B thyroid function tests will be uninterpretable while he is taking amiodarone

C amiodarone normally produces hypothyroidism, and so these symptoms are not likely to be related to amiodarone therapy

D amiodarone should be stopped at once

E If carbimazole alone is not effective, then surgery is indicated

F a positive thyroid-stimulating antibody test would suggest that amiodarone therapy was co-incidental in this case

G prednisolone may be required to control symptoms

H thyroid ultrasonography may help clinical decision making

I suppressed uptake on 99 mTc scintigraphy rules out amiodarone as the responsible agent

J suppressive therapy should be stopped as soon as amiodarone is withdrawn to prevent hypothyroidism

Question 219

A 76-year-old woman with type 2 diabetes mellitus is admitted with a reduced Glasgow Coma Score of 11/15. Her blood results show sodium (Na) 156 mmol/l, potassium (K) 3.2 mmol/l, urea 44 mmol/l and glucose 40 mmol/l. She is not acidotic. If Na, K, glucose and urea are measured in mmol/l, and serum osmolality in mOsm/l, which one of the following equations can be used to calculate plasma osmolality?

A Na + K + glucose = serum osmolality

B Na + K + glucose + urea = serum osmolality

C $2 \times$ (Na + K) + urea = serum osmolality

D $2 \times (Na + K) + glucose / urea = serum\ osmolality$

E $2 \times (Na + K) + glucose + urea = serum\ osmolality$

Question 220

A 43-year-old woman is referred to the endocrine clinic with a corrected serum calcium of 1.56 mmol/l that was recently detected when she had cataract surgery. She has no significant past medical history or family history. Her periods are normal and regular. She went through normal schooling and went to college and studied beauty therapy. She does admit to spasm in her hands when she gets anxious but otherwise has no symptoms of chronic hypocalcaemia. She is short in stature, has horizontal ridges on her nails, and Trousseau's sign is positive. There are no other abnormalities. Other laboratory tests show a raised serum phosphate of 2.56 mmol/l and very low (undetectable) levels of parathyroid hormone (PTH). Her serum cortisol measured at 0900 h, thyroid function tests, urea, creatinine and other electrolytes are normal. Which one of the following diagnoses is most likely?

A pseudohypoparathyroidism

B idiopathic (acquired) hypoparathyroidism

C pseudopseudohypoparathyroidism

D autoimmune hypoparathyroidism (polyglandular auto-immune syndrome type 1)

E chronic renal failure with secondary hyperparathyroidism

Question 221

A 45-year-old man is referred with severe tiredness, frontal headache and lack of libido. He has a bi-temporal hemianopia. Which one of the following results would NOT be consistent with the presence of a pituitary adenoma?

A low insulin-like growth factor-1 (IGF-1) levels

B high prolactin levels

C high follicle-stimulating hormone (FSH) and luteinising hormone (LH) levels with a low testosterone level

D secondary hypothyroidism

E poor (sub-normal) cortisol response to a short synacthen test

Question 222

A 78-year-old man is admitted weak and unable to stand after vomiting for several days. His plasma sodium concentration is 123 mmol/l and his urinary sodium concentration is 8 mmol/l. What is the likely cause of his hyponatraemia?

A syndrome of inappropriate antidiuresis (SIADH)

B diuretic treatment

C loss of sodium in vomit

D hypovolaemic stimulation of ADH release

E Addison's disease

Question 223

A surgical house officer notices that a patient admitted for elective cholecystectomy looks as if they might be acromegalic. They ask you what the best way to establish the diagnosis is. You answer:

A oral glucose tolerance test

B CT scan pituitary fossa

C random growth hormone level

D insulin tolerance test

E lateral skull radiograph

Question 224

A 58-year-old woman presents with symptoms suggestive of bilateral carpal tunnel syndrome. You suspect that she has acromegaly and refer her to the endocrine clinic for further evaluation. Which of the following findings would support this diagnosis?

A random growth hormone (GH) level of 6 mU/l

B GH nadir of 1.0 mU/l during an oral glucose tolerance test (OGTT)

C elevated insulin-like growth factor 1 (IGF-1) level

D left homonymous hemianopia on formal visual field testing

E elevated gonadotrophin (FSH, LH) levels

Question 225

A 54-year-old woman is diagnosed as having acromegaly. She asks you what treatment the endocrinologist, who she is seeing next week, is likely to recommend in the first instance. You answer:

A radiotherapy

B surgery

C octreotide (or other somatostatin analogue)

D bromocriptine (or other dopamine antagonist)

E a growth hormone receptor antagonist

Question 226

A 56-year-old woman is referred following partial thyroidectomy for a goitre that was giving her cosmetic concerns. She says that she is always tired and feels rather cold and weak. Examination does not reveal any gross abnormality: there is no papilloedema or visual field or eye movement defects. Blood tests show TSH 0.9 mU/l (normal range [NR] 0.4 to 4.0 mU/l), free T4 7 pmol/l (NR 10 to 20 pmol/l) and prolactin 4654 mU/l (normal up to 450 mU/l). Which of the following do you think is most important at this stage?

A commence cabergoline without any delay

B urgent short tetracosactide (Synacthen) test and review

C commence thyroxine at low dose and increase gradually

D organise MRI scan of the pituitary gland

E repeat thyroid function test before any further action.

Question 227

A 42-year-old man has proven growth hormone deficiency following pituitary surgery for pituitary adenoma. He is hyperlipidaemic with a family history of ischaemic heart disease. He complains that he has lost his energy and that he is unable to work out in the gym as he used to. Other pituitary axes are either normal or adequately replaced and he is interested in a trial of growth hormone therapy. Which one of the following statements is true?

A he should be commenced on growth hormone as there is evidence that it will reduce his risk of cardiovascular mortality and morbidity.

B he should not commence on growth hormone as it may adversely affect his lipid profile

C treatment with growth hormone may improve his lipid profile and exercise tolerance

D growth hormone treatment is contraindicated due to the risk of re-growth of his pituitary tumour

E growth hormone therapy is important to reduce his risk of osteoporotic fracture

Question 228

As medical registrar on call you are fast bleeped to the ophthalmology clinic to see a 44-year-old woman who has collapsed. She had been referred urgently to the ophthalmologists by her general practitioner after developing a severe frontal headache with nausea and double vision whilst at work. Her past history is remarkable only for migraines, hypothyroidism and mild asthma. She takes hormone replacement therapy and thyroxine as her only regular medications. Before collapsing the ophthalmologist had established that she had an almost complete right third nerve palsy with a left sixth nerve palsy in addition. The discs were rather pale. On examination now she is barely conscious with a pulse rate of 130/min and blood pressure of 70/40 mmHg despite 500 ml of intravenous colloid. There is no evidence of haemorrhage and the abdomen is soft. A further litre of intravenous colloid fails to improve the situation substantially. Which one of the following diagnoses is most likely?

A subarachnoid haemorrhage complicated by a sympathetic storm

B ophthalmoplegic migraine complicated by a vasovagal collapse

C cavernous sinus thrombosis with raised intracranial pressure

D pituitary haemorrhage with secondary hypotensive shock

E phaeochromocytoma crisis with midbrain infarction

Question 229

A 66-year-old woman has been diagnosed with polymyalgia rheumatica and commenced on long-term steroid therapy. Looking at her chest radiograph, it seems likely that she may already have osteoporosis. Which one of the following steps would you take?

A arrange out-patient DEXA scan and treat if she has osteoporosis

B commence anti-resorptive therapy, e.g. alendronate

C advise her to take high calcium diet and exercise regularly

D start her on hormone replacement therapy (HRT)

E consider antiresorptive therapy only if steroids are continued beyond 2 years

Question 230

An 82-year-old woman is admitted having sustained a hip fracture. Two years ago she sustained a wrist fracture. On examination she has bilateral cataracts and reduced visual acuity. She has been on prednisolone 5 mg/d for 8 years for polymyalgia but takes no other regular medication and has not seen a doctor for 2 years. Which one of the following statements about corticosteroid induced osteoporosis is correct?

A corticosteroids increase osteoblastic activity

B corticosteroids increase bone mass

C corticosteroids reduce intestinal calcium absorption

D corticosteroids increase circulating sex steroid levels

E corticosteroid induced osteoporosis is greatest 12 months after starting treatment

Question 231

A 65-year-old woman has Paget's disease. She has increasing bone pain and deformity in the right femur. Serum alkaline phosphatase is raised. Aside from appropriate opioid analgaesia, the correct treatment is:

A add a non-steroidal anti-inflammatory drug

B subcutaneous calcitonin injection

C radiograph of right femur and IV pamidronate infusion

D oral alendronate

E radiograph of right femur and orthopaedic referral

Question 232

A 57-year-old woman with a long history of depressive illness is referred to the endocrine clinic for further investigation of hypercalcaemia (corrected serum calcium level 2.75 mmol/l, normal range 2.1–2.5) that was discovered incidentally. Which of the following drugs is most likely to be of relevance to her current metabolic disturbance?

A citalopram

B haloperidol

C lithium

D venlafaxine

E amitriptyline

Question 233

A 67-year-old woman is admitted following a fall. She is known to be hypertensive and is on treatment with an angiotensin-converting enzyme (ACE) inhibitor. She has chronic renal failure that is presumed to be secondary to hypertension. Routine bloods show sodium 136 mmol/l, potassium 5.2 mmol/l, urea 20.1 mmol/l, creatinine 363 μmol/l, corrected calcium 2.80 mmol/l, phosphate 1.9 mmol/l. The serum parathyroid hormone (PTH) level is 65.5 pmol/l (normal < 5.5 pmol/l). The most likely diagnosis is:

A primary hyperparathyroidism

B secondary hyperparathyroidism

C tertiary hyperparathyroidism

D pseudohypoparathyroidism

E hypercalcaemia secondary to exogenous replacement therapy

Question 234

A 16-year-old boy presents with short stature. He had a normal birth and normal growth and development until about the age of 11 years when he started to fall behind his peers. He is otherwise well. General examination is normal except that he is pre-pubertal (testes 3 ml, Tanner stage G1, P1) with height below the 3rd centile. His bone age is 4 years behind his chronological age. His mid-parental height is on the 50th centile. The likely diagnosis is:

A growth hormone deficiency

B Kleinfelter's syndrome

C Kallman's syndrome

D constitutional delayed puberty

E coeliac disease

Question 235

A 38-year-old man presents with recurrent 'funny turns'. During one of these he is found to have a blood glucose concentration of 1.6 mmol/l. A clever pre-registration house officer sends a concurrent serum sample to the biochemistry laboratory: this is found to contain insulin, but C-peptide levels are low. This means that hypoglycaemia is likely to have been caused by:

A endogenous insulin, e.g. produced by an insulinoma

B consumption of an oral hypoglycaemic agent

C liver disease

D starvation

E exogenous insulin, e.g. self-administration

Question 236

A frail 79-year-old woman has a toxic adenoma of the thyroid that has failed to respond to radioactive iodine given 8 months ago. She remains on carbimazole 20 mg/d and her latest thyroid function test show TSH 0.3 mU/l (normal range 0.4–4.0 mU/l), free T4 22 pmol/l (10–20 pmol/l) and free T3 6.3 pmol/l (3–5.5 pmol/l). What would be the most appropriate line of action?

A leave her on carbimazole indefinitely

B block and replace (use high dose carbimazole to block and replace with thyroxine)

C change carbimazole to propylthiouracil

D refer her for a second dose of radioactive iodine

E refer her to surgeons for thyroidectomy

Nephrology

Nick C Fluck, Philip Kalra, Patrick H Maxwell
(Editor) **and Chris A O'Callaghan**

Nephrology

Answers are on pp. 145–149.

Question 237

A 38-year-old man is crushed when his tractor overturns. He subsequently develops renal failure. Figure 31 shows his arm. Which of the following sets of test results would you expect in this scenario? Note normal range for serum potassium is 3.5–5 mmol/l and for creatine kinase is 25–195 U/l.

A urine stick test—protein 3+, blood 0; serum potassium 5.0 mmol/l; serum creatine kinase 500 U/l

B urine stick test—protein 0, blood 2+; serum potassium 5.0 mmol/l; serum creatine kinase 500 U/l

C urine stick test—protein 0, blood 2+; serum potassium 5.0 mmol/l; serum creatine kinase 5000 U/l

D urine stick test—protein 3+, blood 3+; serum potassium 7.0 mmol/l; serum creatine kinase 50,000 U/l

E urine stick test—protein 1+, blood 3+; serum potassium 3.0 mmol/l; serum creatine kinase 5000 U/l

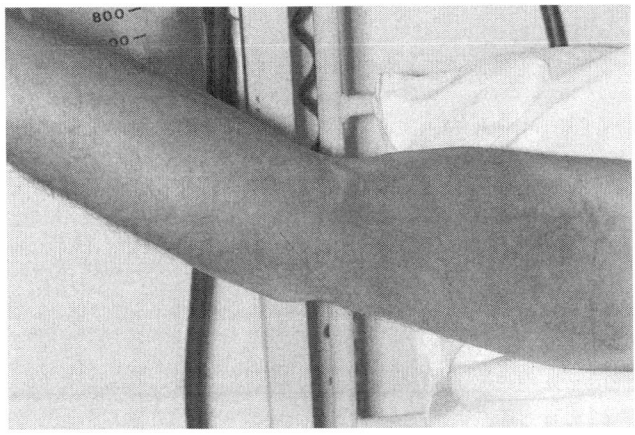

Fig. 31 Question 237.

Question 238

A 58-year-old man with known Wegener's granulomatosis presents with breathlessness that has been getting worse over the last two weeks. He has been feeling a bit feverish, but has not had chest pains, shivers or rigors, and he has not coughed anything up. Prednisolone 5 mg od, azathioprine 150 mg od and ranitidine 150 mg bd are

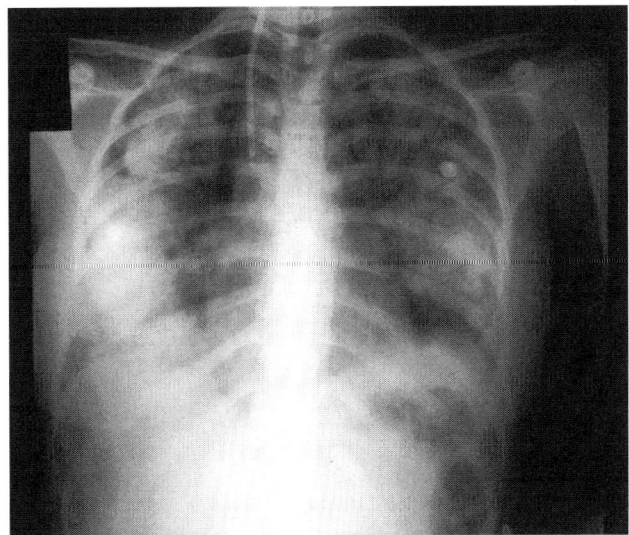

Fig. 32 Question 238.

his only regular medications. On examination he looks very unwell. He is cool and shut down peripherally, cyanosed centrally, and has pulse 130/min (regular) and blood pressure 100/70 mmHg. There are crackles throughout both lung fields. His chest radiograph is shown (see Figure 32). Aside from providing appropriate respiratory and circulatory support, which of the management strategies listed below would be best?

A urgently check titre of anti-neutrophil cytoplasmic antibodies (ANCA), sputum culture, blood culture. Review immediately results available

B urgently organise bronchoscopy and lavage/lung biopsy. Review immediately results available

C urgently check titre of anti-neutrophil cytoplasmic antibodies (ANCA), sputum culture, blood culture. Start treatment for acute relapse of Wegener's pending results

D urgently organise bronchoscopy and lavage/lung biopsy. Start treatment for acute relapse of Wegener's pending results

E start treatment for severe pneumonia and for acute relapse of Wegener's

Question 239

A 66-year-old man presents with a month of malaise, arthralgia and increasing breathlessness. Admission to hospital is precipitated by an episode of haemoptysis. On examination he looks unwell and has a purpuric rash over his trunk. Stick testing of his urine shows proteinuria 3+ and haematuria 2+. Routine blood tests reveal renal failure with serum creatinine of about 600 μmol/l. Some serological tests are performed, also a renal biopsy (see Figure 33) that reveals a condition that affects some glomeruli, but not others, and is patchy in the way that it affects those glomeruli that are affected. The histological diagnosis is:

A focal glomerulonephritis

B focal, segmental glomerulonephritis

C focal, segmental, necrotizing glomerulonephritis

D focal, proliferative glomerulonephritis

E proliferative glomerulonephritis

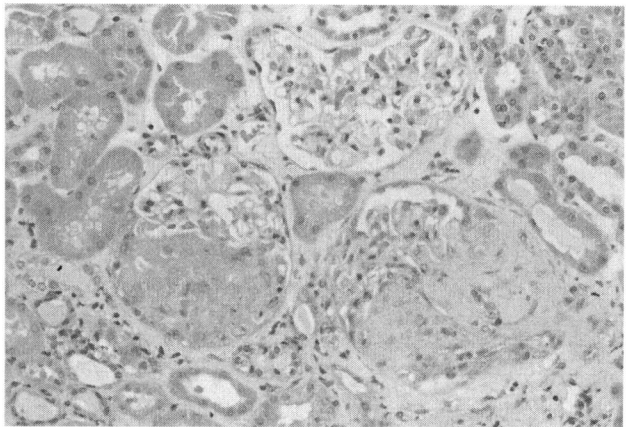

Fig. 33 Question 239.

Question 240

A 69-year-old man with hypertension is found to be hypokalaemic. Which two of the following could NOT account for these findings?

A treatment with a thiazide diuretic

B renal artery stenosis

C Addison's disease

D steroid treatment

E accelerated phase hypertension

F Conn's syndrome

G hypertension treated with spironolactone

H Cushing's disease

I treatment with bumetanide

J activation of the renin-angiotensin system

Question 241

A 60-year-old man presents with non-specific malaise, weight loss, backache and renal impairment. The patient is convinced he has cancer, but there is no evidence of this

on physical examination. His breathing is comfortable and his chest is clear. Urinalysis is negative for protein and blood. Serum electrolytes are normal, but creatinine is 420 μmol/l and C-reactive protein is 30 mg/l (NR <5). Renal ultrasound shows bilateral pelvicalyceal dilatation with good preservation of renal cortical thickness, the prostate is slightly enlarged and the bladder empties completely on micturition. Which two of the following statements are true?

A the patient's GFR is likely to be about 60 ml/min

B computerised tomography would be a useful investigation

C once obstruction is relieved he may be polyuric for several days

D following treatment the chance of the creatinine returning to the normal range is less than 5%

E a urethral catheter should be inserted to allow accurate monitoring of urinary output

F initial treatment should be with three daily doses of 500 mg methylprednisolone

G percutaneous nephrostomies would be a reasonable long-term treatment for his obstructive uropathy

H the patient can be reassured that the most likely diagnosis is probably retroperitoneal fibrosis and that he does not have any form of cancer

I if the diagnosis is retroperitoneal fibrosis, surgical intervention will be necessary

J the immediate priority is to arrange haemodialysis

Question 242

A 68-year-old man receiving regular haemodialysis for chronic renal failure of unknown cause has the following blood test results: sodium 133 mmol/l, potassium 5.1 mmol/l, calcium 1.95 mmol/l and phosphate 1.98 mmol/l. Which two of the following medications are most appropriate to correct these abnormalities?

A sodium pamidronate

B calcium resonium

C 1-alpha hydroxycholecalciferol

D prednisolone

E ergocalciferol

F erythropoietin

G calcium carbonate

H aluminium hydroxide

I alendronate sodium

J sodium bicarbonate

Question 243

During a routine medical check a 27-year-old man who is taking no medication is found to have a blood pressure of

180/97 mmHg and a low serum potassium concentration. His urine contains a trace of protein on dipstick analysis. Which of the following diagnoses is most likely?

A minimal change nephropathy

B primary hyperaldosteronism

C mesangiocapillary glomerulonephritis

D primary hyperparathyroidism

E pseudohypoaldosteronism

Question 244

A 40-year-old man with a 25-year history of diabetes treated with insulin is found to have 2 g proteinuria per 24 hours, haemoglobin 10.5 g/dl, albumen 30 g/l, calcium 2.0 mmol/l, phosphate 1.8 mmol/l, creatinine 250 μmol/l, cholesterol 7 mmol/l. He has significant peripheral oedema. Blood pressure is 135/85 mm Hg. HbA1C is 9.5%. In order to preserve renal function, which of the following do you consider most important?

A strict restriction of dietary phosphate

B commence a loop diuretic

C commence an HMG CoA reductase inhibitor

D commence an angiotensin converting enzyme inhibitor

E greatly improved diabetic control aiming for HbA1c < 7.2%

Question 245

A 37-year-old man, a type I diabetic for six years, presents with a rising serum creatinine concentration. This has been increasing over the last two years, during which time proteinuria has increased from 1+ on stick testing to 12 g/day. On examination he is oedematous and there is mild background diabetic retinopathy but no neuropathy. His blood pressure is mildly elevated at 145/95 mmHg. This is not typical of diabetic nephropathy because:

A onset of renal problems too soon after diagnosis of type I diabetes mellitus

B patients under 40 years of age do not get renal diabetic complications

C significant hypertension is invariable in diabetic nephropathy

D proliferative retinopathy is always seen with significant diabetic renal disease

E diabetic nephropathy rarely causes the nephrotic syndrome

Question 246

A 32-year-old man presents to his general practitioner with a non-specific history of malaise. On examination he

looks pale and blood pressure is 170/100 mmHg, but there are no other abnormal findings. Initial investigations identify significant anaemia with fragmentation on the blood film and low platelets. A clotting screen is normal. Biochemical tests reveal significant renal dysfunction with serum creatinine 260 μmol/l. What is the most likely diagnosis?

A thrombotic thrombocytopenic purpura (TTP)

B haemolytic uraemic syndrome

C malignant hypertension

D disseminated intravascular coagulation

E systemic vasculitis

Question 247

A 53-year-old-man is found to have a blood pressure of 185/95 mmHg at a routine medical check. His general practitioner checks his electrolytes and renal function, which are normal, and then starts him on an angiotensin-converting enzyme inhibitor. A week later these blood tests are repeated. Which one of the following is NOT a possible direct consequence of starting an angiotensin-converting enzyme (ACE) inhibitor?

A a rise in plasma potassium

B a rise in plasma creatinine

C a rise in plasma sodium

D a fall in glomerular filtration rate

E a fall in aldosterone production

Question 248

A 19-year-old army recruit presents with acute renal failure. Which of the following features is NOT consistent with a diagnosis of rhabdomyolysis?

A elevated plasma creatine kinase level

B anuria

C elevated plasma creatinine

D blood and red cell casts in the urine

E hyperkalaemia

Question 249

A 45-year-old man with adult polycystic kidney disease and plasma creatinine 300 μmol/l is found to have serum potassium 5.1 mmol/l, calcium 2.25 mmol/l, albumin 40 g/l, phosphate 1.65 mmol/l, and PTH 20 pmol/l (NR 1.1–6.8). He has already seen a specialist dietician for advice concerning potassium and phosphate intake. He is currently taking an angiotensin-converting enzyme (ACE)-inhibitor for hypertension and a proton pump inhibitor for reflux oesophagitis. Which of the following statements is true?

A he should be commenced on alfacalcidol 0.5 mcg od, to correct deficiency of active vitamin D and suppress parathyroid hormone (PTH)
B an appropriate treatment would be calcium acetate 1 g bd to be taken with meals
C aluminium hydroxide should be the first choice if a phosphate binder is prescribed
D parathyroidectomy should be considered, especially if he is keen on having a renal transplant in the future
E sevelamer (Renagel) should be used here in preference to other phosphate binders

Question 250

A 17-year-old boy presents with a short history of sudden onset of severely swollen ankles. He is otherwise well, and urinalysis shows 3+ proteinuria. A urinary collection shows that he is excreting 6 g protein per 24 hours. The serum albumen concentration is reduced, but serum creatinine is in the normal range. What is the most likely underlying diagnosis?
A thin membrane nephropathy
B membranous nephropathy
C minimal change nephrotic syndrome
D IgA nephropathy
E mesangiocapillary glomerulonephritis

Question 251

A 52-year-old man presents with acute colicky pain that radiates from his left loin to his left groin and is associated with nausea and vomiting. A plain abdominal radiograph is unremarkable, but ultrasound examination demonstrates pelvi-calyceal dilatation and the presence of several masses that cast acoustic shadows in the left renal pelvis. The most likely diagnosis is:
A adult polycystic kidney disease
B papillary necrosis
C cystine renal stones
D uric acid renal stones
E calcium oxalate renal stones

Question 252

A 22-year-old woman presents with recurrent symptoms of urinary frequency and dysuria associated with cloudy urine. These settle rapidly with courses of antibiotics. Which one of the following would NOT be a recognised strategy for trying to prevent recurrence?
A long-term prophylaxis with trimethoprim 100 mg at night
B regular drinking of cranberry juice

C practice of double micturition
D advice to void the bladder before and after sexual activity
E wash using a shower rather than a bath

Question 253

A 30-year-old man, a haemodialysis patient with diabetic nephropathy, has a serum calcium of 2.9 mmol/l and phosphate of 2.5 mmol/l. Serum alkaline phosphatase and albumen are within their normal ranges and PTH is at the lower end of the normal laboratory range. The patient's current medication includes alfacalcidol each day and calcium acetate as a phosphate binder before each meal. Select the most appropriate statement.
A phosphate restriction in the diet should be reinforced, a change of phosphate binder may be necessary and alfacalcidol should be reduced or stopped
B the dialysate calcium should be lowered to return the calcium to the normal range
C the calcium acetate dose should be reduced to return the calcium to the normal range
D the patient has autonomous hyperparathyroidism
E these values are satisfactory for a haemodialysis patient

Question 254

A 58-year-old man with end stage renal failure secondary to adult polycystic kidney disease receives regular haemodialysis three times per week. He is troubled by gout. Which of the following treatments is UNLIKELY to prove effective?
A allopurinol
B prednisolone
C colchicine
D probenecid
E increased dialysis

Question 255

You are providing a seminar for patients approaching the need for renal replacement therapy. A group of patients contemplating starting continuous ambulatory peritoneal dialysis (CAPD) ask you about medical contraindications to this modality. Which of the following is NOT a relative contraindication to CAPD treatment?
A previous perforated diverticular disease and sigmoid colectomy
B bilateral inguinal herniae
C diabetes mellitus
D severe chronic obstructive pulmonary disease
E arthritis mutilans

Question 256

A 36-year-old man who received a renal transplant 18 months ago is admitted with a history of pyrexia and weight loss, the physical finding of cervical lymphadenopathy, and laboratory tests showing rising serum creatinine, anaemia and abnormal liver enzymes. His immediate post transplant period had been complicated by an episode of cellular rejection and one of vascular rejection, treated with methylprednisolone and antithymocyte globulin (ATG) respectively. What is the most likely diagnosis?

A cytomegalovirus (CMV) disease

B acute cellular rejection

C chronic allograft rejection

D post transplant lymphoproliferative disorder

E tuberculosis

Question 257

A 28-year-old woman received a kidney transplant from her brother. Six weeks after transplantation she was admitted with epigastric pain, vomiting and fever. Blood tests demonstrated markedly abnormal liver function tests with a hepatocellular pattern of derangement. Which of the following medications had been given at the time of transplantation to try to prevent this complication?

A aspirin

B ranitidine

C nifedipine

D co-trimoxazole (Septrin)

E aciclovir

Question 258

A 46-year-old man presents with a 23-year history of lithium carbonate therapy for bipolar affective disorder. He is polyuric (11 litres/day) and has 2 grams/day of proteinuria. His GFR is 47-mls/min/1.73 m^2. Blood pressure is raised at 150/100 mmHg. He has a renal biopsy. What would be typical findings?

A IgA glomerulonephritis

B crescentic glomerulonephritis

C renal vasculitis

D focal glomerulosclerosis and interstitial nephritis

E granulomata

Question 259

A 64-year-old woman is referred to the renal outpatient clinic for investigation of abnormal renal function, detected after she consulted her general practitioner following an episode of macroscopic haematuria. She has a 20-year history of low back pain treated with a combination of painkillers. Ultrasound examination identifies two smallish irregularly-shaped kidneys. Which of the following is the most likely diagnosis?

A IgA nephropathy

B myeloma kidney

C analgesic nephropathy

D acute interstitial nephritis

E membranous nephropathy

Question 260

Which of the following tests do you think would be the most appropriate in supporting a diagnosis of reflux nephropathy in a 40-year-old man with plasma creatinine 540 μmole/litre, 2.5 g proteinuria per 24 hours, and a childhood history of repeated urinary tract infections?

A micturating cystogram

B renal ultrasound

C intravenous urography

D computerized tomography with intravenous contrast

E isotopic imaging with 99 mTc-DTPA

Question 261

A 56-year-old woman with a long and complicated past medical history presents with malaise. Blood tests reveal that she has significant renal impairment, with serum creatinine 417 μmol/l compared to a value of 108 μmol/l taken at a routine visit to a rheumatological clinic three months previously. A variety of tests of blood and urine do not establish a diagnosis, ultrasound examination shows two normal-sized unobstructed kidneys, and she proceeds to renal biopsy that reveals acute interstitial nephritis. Which of her many drugs is most likely to have been responsible?

A paracetamol

B co-proxamol

C enalapril

D atorvastatin

E omeprazole

Rheumatology and clinical immunology

Khalid Binymin, Hilary J Longhurst,
Siraj A Misbah *(Editor)* and
Neil Snowden

Rheumatology and Clinical Immunology

Answers are on pp. 149–152.

Question 262

Consider Table 1. A 38-year-old woman with a history of perennial rhinitis undergoes skin prick testing, which one of the following patterns of response is most likely to be hers?

A pattern 1
B pattern 2
C pattern 3
D pattern 4
E pattern 5

Question 263

An 18-year-old man is under investigation for Crohn's disease because of chronic perianal sepsis, with fistula formation after drainage of an abscess. He presents with fever. His CT scan is shown (Figure 34). His 4-year-old brother was recently treated for a similar condition. What is the likely diagnosis?

A familial Crohn's disease
B inherited complement deficiency
C inherited neutrophil killing defect
D inherited cytokine/cytokine receptor deficiency
E inherited T-cell deficiency

Question 264

A 36-year-old man presents with an 8-week history of sinusitis and arthralgia. The sinusitis has not improved with prolonged antibiotic treatment. His serum CRP is markedly raised at 125 mg/l (reference range 0–10 mg/l). The appearances of his paranasal sinuses on CT scan are shown (Figure 35a), also the results of an indirect immuno-fluorescence test of his serum using human ethanol-

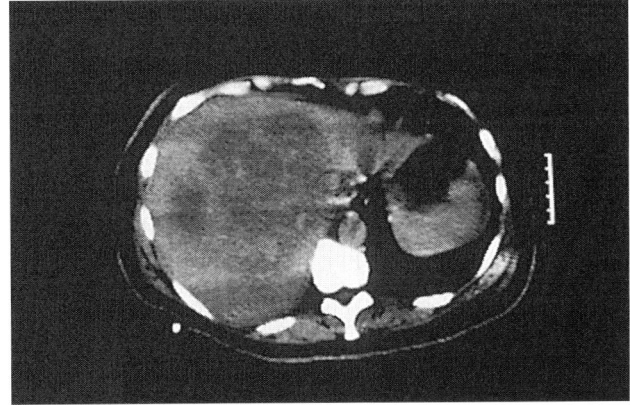

Fig. 34 Question 263. (With permission from Bannister BA, Begg NT, Gillespie SH. *Infectious Disease*, 2nd edn. Oxford: Blackwell Science, 2000.)

fixed neutrophils as a substrate (Figure 35b). What is the likely diagnosis?

A systemic lupus erythematosus
B diffuse cutaneous systemic sclerosis
C polyarteritis nodosa
D microscopic polyangiitis
E Wegener's granulomatosis

Question 265

A 63-year-old man with no previous history of arthritis presents with a painful, swollen knee joint. You are uncertain of the diagnosis and perform diagnostic aspiration. Which one of the fluids described in Table 2 would be compatible with the diagnosis of pseudogout, or would none of them?

A fluid A
B fluid B
C fluid C

Table 1 Question 262: skin prick test results – the diameter of the weal is shown (in millimetres).

	Diluent (negative) (mm)	Histamine (mm)	Grass pollen (mm)	House dust mite (mm)	Latex (mm)
1	1	7	0	4	0
2	0	4	1 + 8 of erythema	0	0
3	0	1	0	2	0
4	5	7	3	4	3
5	0	6	4	0	0

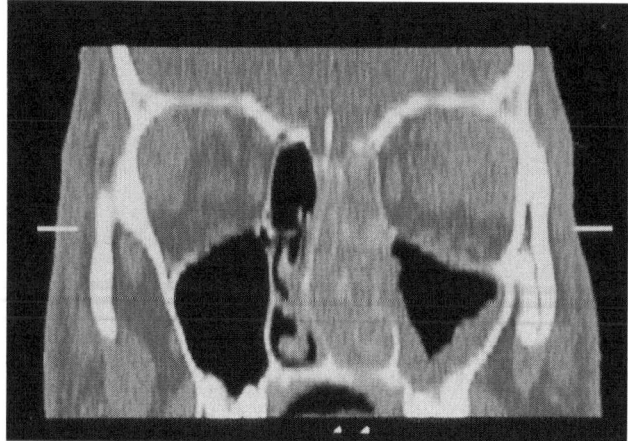

(a)

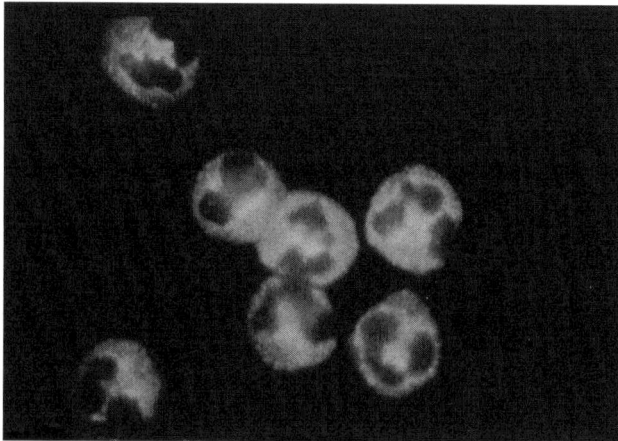

(b)

Fig. 35 Question 264.

D fluid D
E none of the fluids described

Question 266
A 75-year-old woman presents with a 24-hour history of a painful swollen right knee. She feels generally unwell and

has a temperature of 38.1°C. She has had minor pain and stiffness in both knees for many years. Select the most likely diagnosis, and the diagnosis that requires rapid exclusion.

A gout
B rheumatoid arthritis
C primary generalised osteoarthritis
D pseudogout
E reactive arthritis
F osteonecrosis
G haemarthrosis
H avascular necrosis
I septic arthritis
J haemochromatosis

Question 267
A 34-year-old man presents with severe low back pain, which has forced him to stop work as a bus driver. He has had back pain on and off for many years, on occasion with right-sided sciatica. The pain used to be helped by rest, but is now present more or less all the time and is stopping him from sleeping properly. The most likely diagnosis is:

A mechanical back pain
B ankylosing spondylitis
C myeloma
D osteoporosis
E osteoarthritis

Question 268
A 20-year-old man with common variable antibody deficiency presents to the Accident and Emergency department with a 3-day history of cough productive of green sputum. His temperature is 37.5°C, pulse 84/min, respiratory rate 12/min, and breath sounds are vesicular. The chest radiograph is unremarkable. Which two immediate actions do you recommend?

A prescribe a 14-day course of antibiotics
B prescribe nebulised salbutamol

Table 2 Question 265: synovial fluid analyses.

	Fluid A	Fluid B	Fluid C	Fluid D
Macroscopic appearance	Clear	Turbid	Turbid	Turbid
Microscopy	<1000 cells/mm³	50 000 cells/mm³, mainly neutrophils	60 000 cells/mm³, mainly neutrophils	125 000 cells/mm³, mainly neutrophils
	No crystals	Needle-shaped crystals	No crystals	Large numbers
Culture	No organisms	No organisms	No organisms	Gram-positive cocci
	Sterile	Sterile	Sterile	*Staphylococcus aureus* +++

C give an infusion of intravenous immunoglobulin

D take a sputum sample to look for acid fast bacilli

E prescribe a 5-day course of antibiotics

F check his serum immunoglobulin levels

G choose an antibiotic regimen suitable for possible pseudomonas infection

H order a high resolution CT scan

I take a sputum sample for culture

J prescribe a 28-day course of antibiotics

Question 269

A 27-year-old woman has a 6-year history of systemic lupus erythematosus (SLE) treated with azathioprine, hydroxychloroquine and prednisolone. She presents with a 2-week history of slowly worsening severe pain and restriction of the right hip. Which two of the following diagnoses seem most likely?

A gout

B flare of systemic lupus erythematosus (SLE)

C secondary osteoarthritis

D Perthe's disease

E septic arthritis

F secondary fibromyalgia

G irritable hip

H osteoporotic fracture of femoral neck

I avascular necrosis of the femoral head

J slipped upper femoral epiphysis

Question 270

The parents of a 10-year-old asthmatic boy with peanut allergy are concerned about the risk of future anaphylaxis if he were to inadvertently ingest peanuts. Which of the following features is the single most important predictor of anaphylaxis in this situation?

A level of peanut-specific IgE in his serum

B strength of positive skin test response to peanut

C poorly controlled asthma

D previous steroid therapy

E family history of nut allergy

Question 271

A 34-year-old woman presents to your clinic complaining of cold hands, particularly in the winter months. On examination she has cold dusky hands and a petechial rash. Investigations are as follows: Hb 10.9 g/dL; WBC 4.2×10^9/L; platelets 407×10^9/L; urea and electrolytes – normal; liver function tests – normal; albumin 36 g/L; globulin 90 g/L; Protein electrophoresis – polyclonal increase

in gammaglobulins; antinuclear antibodies present (1/160, speckled pattern); complement – C3 0.79 (NR 0.75–1.25), C4 < 0.04 (NR 0.14–0.6). Which one of the following statements is true?

A active systemic lupus erythematous (SLE) is unlikely if DNA antibodies are present

B a blood sample sent to the lab on ice may show cryoglobulins

C Sjögren's syndrome is unlikely if rheumatoid factor is present

D Sjögren's syndrome is likely if Ro and La extractable nuclear antigens are present

E hepatitis C is unlikely in this case

Question 272

A 28-year-old man has recently been discharged from hospital after treatment for pneumococcal pneumonia. He has had repeated courses of antibiotics for sinus, ear and lower respiratory tract infections, and had sinus surgery the previous year. He is a life-long non-smoker and is not on medication. His blood count prior to discharge was normal. In the absence of further clues in the history or examination, which single blood test is the most important?

A HIV antibody test

B pneumococcal antibodies

C immunoglobulin levels

D liver function tests

E IgG subclass levels

Question 273

A 20-year-old woman presents with sudden onset of swelling of the lips and tongue. She also has attacks of abdominal pain and vomiting, which her mother confirms have occurred intermittently over many years. A brother and older sister have the same disorder. Which one of the following statements about this disease is accurate?

A it has sex-linked inheritance

B animal allergen is often identified in the house

C serum C4 levels are often low

D antinuclear antibodies (ANA) is often positive

E raised IgE helps differentiate it from other immune disorders

Question 274

A 60-year-old accountant complains of recurrent attacks of exquisite pain and swelling in the left big toe. Which of the following conditions is NOT likely to be associated with this disorder?

A chronic alcoholism

B obesity

C rheumatoid arthritis

D diabetes mellitus

E diuretic therapy

Question 275

A 65-year-old woman with a mitral valve replacement presents to the Accident and Emergency department with pyrexia and fainting. She is unwell, hypotensive, anaemic and pyrexial. She has a vague history of suffering from a reaction to penicillin in her childhood. After taking blood cultures she is started on broad-spectrum antibiotics. Cardiac valvular vegetations are seen on echocardiography and her blood grows methicillin-sensitive *Staphylococci*. The microbiologist suggests naficillin as the most appropriate antibiotic, but is concerned that she may have an allergy to beta lactam-based antibiotics. Which of the following is most appropriate to investigate the history of possible penicillin allergy?

A serum tryptase

B skin prick test to penicillin

C serum penicillin specific IgE

D patch test to penicillin

E serum IgE

Question 276

A 30-year-old female nurse presents with a 3-month history of Raynaud's phenomenon. Clinical examination reveals cold hands but no other evidence of connective tissue disease. Which of the following tests is most helpful in determining future progression to systemic connective tissue disease?

A positive anti-mitochondrial antibody

B positive anti-gastric parietal cell antibody

C positive smooth muscle antibody

D positive anti-nuclear antibody

E positive rheumatoid factor

Question 277

A 28-year-old woman presents with fatigue and extreme tiredness. Physical examination reveals facial skin rash and tenderness across the small joints of the hands. She is concerned that she might have systemic lupus erythematosus (SLE). Which one of the following tests will virtually exclude the diagnosis of SLE as cause for her symptoms if it is NEGATIVE?

A antinuclear antibody (ANA)

B anti-double stranded DNA

C anti-Sm antibodies

D anti-histone antibodies

E anti-Ro/SS-A antibodies

Question 278

A 66-year-old woman has a 15-year history of deforming rheumatoid arthritis (RA) for which she takes D-penicillamine. Two weeks ago she noticed increased difficulty in climbing stairs and three days before admission she was unable to comb her hair or feed herself. Neurological assessment reveals weakness in arms and legs. Both plantars are upgoing. Which one of the following tests is most likely to provide the diagnosis?

A plain radiograph of the cervical spine

B electromyography (EMG)

C nerve conduction study (NCS)

D isotope bone scan

E magnetic resonance imaging (MRI) of the cervical spine

Question 279

A 35-year-old man is referred for investigation of recurrent infection. He has had frequent respiratory tract infections for the past 5 years, requiring 4–5 courses of antibiotics each winter. A month previously he was admitted with pneumococcal pneumonia, and two months prior to that he had sinus surgery. Which of the following conditions is NOT in the differential diagnosis?

A antibody deficiency

B HIV infection

C bronchiectasis secondary to recurrent infection

D complement C6 deficiency

E smoking 5 cigarettes per day

Question 280

A 19-year-old woman presents with fever and cough. Sputum samples are negative on microscopy for acid fast bacilli, but six weeks later *M. tuberculosis* (MTB) is grown. She completed a course of chemotherapy for pulmonary TB two months previously. Her chest radiograph is unchanged from one taken at this time. Which of the following is the most likely explanation for these findings?

A she has HIV co-infection causing increased susceptibility to mycobacteria

B the organism isolated is a contaminant

C she has been re-infected with a different strain of TB
D she has underlying IFNγ receptor deficiency causing increased susceptibility to mycobacteria
E she has been poorly adherent to therapy and her TB has recurred

Question 281

A 65-year-old woman presents with a 3-month history of recurrent attacks of facial angioedema. Which of the following test results would favour a diagnosis of C1 inhibitor deficiency?
A low complement C3 levels and a normal C4
B low complement C4 levels and a normal C3
C hypergammaglobulinaemia
D hypogammaglobulinaemia
E positive rheumatoid factor

Question 282

A 30-year-old woman develops a systemic reaction characterised by hypotension, bronchospasm and widespread urticaria soon after induction of anaesthesia for cholecystectomy. Which of the following blood test results would suggest that her reaction was associated with mast cell degranulation?
A elevated plasma tryptase
B hypernatraemia
C hypokalaemia
D hypocomplementaemia
E hypergammaglobulinaemia

Question 283

A 50-year-old man gives an 8-month history of episodic, painful soft tissue swellings involving his hands, eyes and lips. There is no temporal relationship to food. Which of the following tests is the most useful?
A skin prick tests to various food allergens
B serum complement
C full blood count (FBC)
D glucose tolerance test
E urinary 5-hydroxyindoleacetic acid

Answers

Clinical Pharmacology

Answer to Question 1
C

Ketoconazole inhibits liver enzymes that metabolise ciclosporin, increasing plasma ciclosporin concentration and potentially leading to nephrotoxicity. Deterioration in renal function could be seen if enalapril is started on a background of renal artery stenosis, but in this case the close relationship between the timing of the course of ketoconazole and the increase in creatinine makes option C the most likely.

Answer to Question 2
A

Clozapine has fewer extrapyramidal adverse effects than older antipsychotics, which is attributed to its relatively low affinity for D2 dopamine receptors. Unlike older antipsychotics, clozapine has relatively high affinity for 5HT receptors and also has little effect on prolactin levels.

Myocarditis and cardiomyopathy have been reported with atypical antipsychotics, with persistent tachycardia an early warning sign. Agranulocytosis is a well-recognized complication of clozapine: patients should be supervised under the Clozaril Patient Monitoring Service.

Answer to Question 3
C

Evidence underpinning the choice of anti-hypertensive therapy in pregnancy is inadequate to make firm recommendations. There are no reports of serious effects with methyldopa following long and extensive use. Calcium antagonists, labetalol and hydralazine are commonly used, particularly for resistant hypertension in the third trimester. However, angiotensin-converting enzyme (ACE)-inhibitors should be avoided because they may cause oligohydramnios, renal failure and intra-uterine death.

Answer to Question 4
A

Drugs such as apomorphine and bromocriptine cause vomiting through peripheral stimulation of the chemoreceptor trigger zone. Worsening of Parkinson's disease

may result from the use of dopamine antagonists, but domperidone is not likely to cross the blood–brain barrier and is therefore the preferred agent in this case. Entacapone is a catechol-O-methyltransferase (COMT) inhibitor that increases levodopa levels, thus worsening nausea and vomiting. Betahistine is used in vertigo.

Answer to Question 5
C

Ciprofloxacin has been associated with arthropathy and cartilage erosions in young animals. Gentamicin needs to be given parenterally and is not suitable for outpatient use, and there is also a risk of fetal nephrotoxicity and ototoxicity. Trimethoprim is a folate antagonist and can increase the risk of neural tube defects. Co-amoxiclav is a combination of amoxycillin and clavulanic acid, and although there is no definite risk of teratogenicity it should not be used unless absolutely necessary. Furthermore, this patient has previously had a rash with penicillin. Although there is a small risk of cross-allergy (10%) with cephalosporins, cefaclor would be the best choice given that the penicillin allergy was relatively mild and not a full-blown anaphylactic reaction.

Answer to Question 6
D

Anti-thyroid drugs can cross the placenta and breast milk, thus causing hypothyroidism in the child. The carbimazole block-and-replace regimen is the worst in this respect, as the carbimazole crosses the placenta but the thyroxine does not. Potassium perchlorate is no longer used in the UK; Lugol's iodine may occasionally be prescribed for patients undergoing thyroid surgery, but causes goitre in infants. Propythiouracil is more highly protein bound and is ionized at pH 7.4, thus making it less likely to cross the placenta or breast milk.

Answer to Question 7
D

Anticholinergic syndrome occurs following overdose with drugs that have prominent anticholinergic activity, including tricyclic antidepressants, antihistamines and atropine. Features include dry, warm, flushed skin, urinary retention, tachycardia, mydriasis (dilated pupils) and agitation. Although physostigmine, a reversible inhibitor of acetylcholinesterase, is effective in treating symptoms, there is a significant risk of cardiac toxicity (bradycardia, AV conduction defects and asystole). Treatment therefore

113

consists of withdrawal of the precipitating drug and supportive care.

Answer to Question 8

C

This man has carbon monoxide (CO) poisoning. Pulse oximeters cannot distinguish between COHb and HbO_2, therefore it is essential to take arterial blood gases and – to make the specific diagnosis – measure the level of CO. It is important to think about prevention: CO alarms are cheap and readily available.

Answer to Question 9

B

Aspirin in excess causes symptoms of nausea, vomiting, headache, confusion and tinnitus or hearing difficulties. Whilst the co-codamol and codeine phosphate could cause confusion, they would not cause the tinnitus. All analgesics taken for a prolonged period of time can lead to an analgesic-induced headache.

Answer to Question 10

A

Reactions to NAC are well recognized and are not related to hypersensitivity. NAC can almost always be safely restarted and the full treatment dose safely administered after symptomatic treatment. Oral methionine may be an alternative but is definitely second line. IV chlorpromazine would make hypotension worse. Withholding treatment and waiting more than 12 hours would expose the patient to risk of liver failure.

Answer to Question 11

A

Rizatriptan is not used as prophylaxis against migraine. It is a 5HT1 agonist and may be useful in the treatment of acute attacks, for which it is available as either tablets or 'melt wafers' that dissolve on the tongue.

Propranolol and pizotifen are licensed for use as prophylaxis against migraine. Pizotifen may cause drowsiness and weight gain. Sodium valproate and amitriptyline are unlicensed for migraine prophylaxis but can be effective in some patients.

Answer to Question 12

C

About 25% of patients who stop their anti-epilepsy treatment will relapse within a year of starting to taper down their medication. The likelihood of seizure is greatest during withdrawal and in the subsequent 6 months. The DVLA recommends that patients should not drive during this period.

Doses of drugs such as carbamazepine, lamotrigine, phenytoin, sodium valproate and vigabatrin should be reduced by about 10% every 2–4 weeks. Barbiturates, benzodiazepines and ethosuximide should be tapered more slowly by reducing dosage by about 10% every 4–8 weeks. Only one drug should be withdrawn at a time, with a period of 1 month between completing withdrawal of one drug and beginning withdrawal of the next. There is no evidence to support the belief that patients become resistant to their original therapy following discontinuation.

Answer to Question 13

A

Vasoactive drugs have limited benefit in treating intermittent claudication. There is modest evidence for the use of drugs such as naftidrofuryl and pentoxifylline, but little benefit from cinnarizine or inositol nicotinate. Simvastatin may be prescribed for patients with peripheral vascular disease who have elevated cholesterol levels, but there is no data on improvements in walking distance.

Answer to Question 14

D

Diazepam has a long half-life, principally because of its active metabolites. Midazolam is short-acting but is only used intravenously. Promethazine is an antihistamine with a 12-hour half-life and may cause daytime sedation. Clomethiazole is less safe in overdose, has dependence potential and is only licensed for sedation in the elderly. Loprazolam is short-acting (half-life 6–12 hours) and would be a reasonable choice in this case.

Answer to Question 15

B

The options for treatment of atrial fibrillation are:
• DC cardioversion if the patient is compromised haemodynamically or has ischaemic cardiac pain
• Digoxin – 1.0–1.5 mg orally in divided doses over 24 hours, but can be given intavenously in emergency (0.25–0.5 mg over 10–20 min, repeated after four to eight hours to total intravenous loading dose of 0.5–1.0 mg)
• 'Medical cardioversion' with amiodarone or flecainide
In this clinical context it is likely that the atrial fibrillation (if new) will revert to sinus rhythm as the woman recovers

from her pneumonia and most physicians would digitalize in preference to the other options described.

Pain Relief and Palliative Care

Answer to Question 16

F, I

The patient requires sedation rather than more analgesia. A stat dose of either midazolam or levomepromazine will allow you to calculate the 24-hour dose needed for the syringe driver.

Answer to Question 17

A, D

Symptoms of opioid withdrawal are often likened to 'cold turkey', i.e. shivering, sweating, lacrimation and rhinorrhea. Patients feel generally unwell and 'fluey' with muscle aches, nausea and vomiting and diarrhoea.

Answer to Question 18

E

Loss of sphincter control can result in faecal incontinence, which is distressing for patients. High dose stimulant laxatives are likely to result in increased faecal incontinence, and co-danthramer can cause rashes if in contact with skin for prolonged periods. A common compromise is to clear the rectum (with manual evacuation or enema), then use low dose laxatives to soften the stool. By using regular enemas, the patient has a predictable bowel movement and a reduced risk of incontinence.

Answer to Question 19

E

In this circumstance it is best to anticipate problems and avoid the development of pain. A syringe driver with the correct dose of diamorphine and 1/6 dose as breakthrough medication is correct.

Answer to Question 20

D

The history suggests that there may be a neuromuscular cause for his symptoms. Another possibility is external compression, but the endoscopy did not show this. Metoclopramide is both an antidopaminergic and a gastrokinetic agent that may improve oesophageal motility.

Answer to Question 21

A

Bulk forming drugs such as fybogel have little to offer in opioid-induced constipation. Senna can cause abdominal cramps. Co-danthramer can cause skin burns in faecal incontinence: this patient is frail and may not be able to clean herself well and is therefore at risk of this most unpleasant complication. Lactulose can cause bowel distension and increased abdominal cramps.

Medicine for the Elderly

Answer to Question 22

D

The liver is enlarged, there are several metastases in it (darker areas at right lateral border and anteriorly), and there is ascites (fluid around the liver, appearing black).

With this clinical history the most likely diagnosis is metastatic colonic carcinoma, but other malignancies that are common in this age group (breast, lung, ovary) should be considered.

Answer to Question 23

E

Her symptoms are compatible with anaemia, and the picture shows glossitis and angular cheilosis. Given the history it is likely that she will have poor diet. Deficiency of iron and/or folate is likely in this context and could explain both anaemia and the appearances shown.

Answer to Question 24

G, I

Benzhexol is an anticholinergic drug with the usual anticholinergic side effects: it is said to be more effective for tremor than other features of Parkinson's. Long-term anticholinergic treatment should not be stopped abruptly as patients can deteriorate significantly. Benzhexol should be avoided in patients with dementia due to its neuropsychiatric side effect profile.

Levodopa combined with a peripheral decarboxylase inhibitor does not cross the blood–brain barrier. It can cause motor fluctuations and dyskinesia, and it may discolour urine and sweat.

Amantadine can cause confusion. Apomorphine is a D1 and D2 receptor agonist. Selegiline is a selective inhibitor of monoamine oxidase type B.

Answer to Question 25

C, F

Rigidity is usually present in Parkinson's disease, but not always, and tremor is absent in 30% of cases. Upper body akinesia must be present to diagnose Parkinson's disease. Cumulative lifetime risk of developing Parkinsonism is estimated at 1 in 40. The diagnosis of Parkinson's disease is entirely clinical. Essential tremor and arteriosclerotic pseudo-parkinsonism are commonly misdiagnosed as Parkinson's disease. In essential tremor there may be secondary cogwheeling but no lead pipe rigidity or true akinesia. Rapid progression would suggest non-idiopathic Parkinsonism.

Answer to Question 26

D

A pressure sore/ulcer develops when persistent pressure on a bony site (e.g. heel, greater trochanter) obstructs capillary blood flow: necrosis of tissue can develop within two hours or less. Early stages include changes in skin temperature (warmth or coolness), altered tissue consistency (boggy or firm), and itching. Later stages include partial or full thickness skin loss and destruction of adjacent tissue. Many predisposing factors have been identified (e.g. sepsis, urinary incontinence, diabetes mellitus, immobility) and there are a range of well-validated tools to identify patients at risk.

The use of support surfaces to redistribute pressure has been shown to improve outcomes and reduce costs. Repositioning the patient at least every two hours is also an important component of prevention/management. Attention to nutrition is important to increase wound healing, particularly in those with protein malnutrition.

Answer to Question 27

D

Many psychiatric drugs should not be stopped precipitously, including selective serotonin reuptake inhibitors (SSRIs) such as paroxetine and benzodiazepines (such as lorazepam). If the dose of these medications needs to be changed, this must be done very slowly, otherwise they can produce an acute withdrawal state with worsening confusion and agitation. The same applies to alcohol. Her family can bring in her usual tipple, so that the nurses can monitor intake, otherwise prescribe chlordiazepoxide in reducing doses.

It is important to check her thyroid-stimulating hormone (TSH) level to ensure she is on the correct dose of thyroxine, but this is unlikely to be the cause of the confusion.

Cimetidine can cause confusion in older people and can safely be stopped. Does she still need ulcer-healing treatment? If so, consider a proton pump inhibitor.

Answer to Question 28

C

Tapering and discontinuation of psychotropic drugs, including benzodiazepines and antidepressants, has been shown to reduce the incidence of falls. Some older people with postural hypotension are asymptomatic. Falls account for 6% of acute hospital admissions.

Reducing the number of medications to 4 or less has been shown to reduce the number of falls in older people.

Answer to Question 29

A

Drugs such as apomorphine and bromocriptine cause vomiting through peripheral stimulation of the chemoreceptor trigger zone. Worsening of Parkinson's disease may result from the use of dopamine antagonists: domperidone is much less likely to cross the blood–brain barrier and is therefore the preferred agent in this case. Entacapone is a catechol-O-methyltransferase (COMT) inhibitor which increases levodopa levels, thus worsening nausea and vomiting. Betahistine is used in vertigo.

Answer to Question 30

D

Incontinence should be managed by institution of simple measures such as regular toileting, bladder re-training (gradually increasing the time between voidings), limitation of fluid intake (typically to 1.5 L/day), treatment of atrophic vaginitis, avoidance of bladder irritants (caffeine, alcohol), improving mobility and access to toilets, and sensible choice of clothing.

If these measures fail to provide relief, then pharmacological treatment is appropriate and all of those listed can be effective in urge incontinence. Oxybutinin, tolterodine and flavoxate are all anticholinergics, and imipramine has anticholinergic action, hence all of these are likely to cause a dry mouth.

Answer to Question 31

C

Stress incontinence describes the involuntary leaking of small amounts of urine on coughing, laughing or exercising. Urge incontinence describes an overwhelming and instant urge to pass urine with involuntary emptying of the bladder. Mixed type incontinence has features of both stress and urge incontinence. Functional incontinence describes the situation where the patient is unable to get to the toilet, perhaps secondary to reduced mobility or confusion.

Answer to Question 32
D

The Barthel Index quantitates performance of basic activities of daily living. Ten activities are assessed: feeding, bathing, grooming, dressing, bowels, bladder, toilet, bed/chair, ambulation, stairs. The maximum score is 20.

Answer to Question 33
E

The Abbreviated Mental Test Score (AMT) asks the following ten questions:
- Age
- Time (to nearest hour)
- Address for recall at the end (e.g. 42 West Street)
- What year is it?
- Name of institution
- Recognition of two persons (e.g. nurse and doctor)
- Date of birth (day and month)
- Year of First World War
- Name of present monarch
- Count backwards from 20 to 1

Answer to Question 34
E

The triad of dementia, urinary incontinence and gait disturbance is classically associated with normal pressure hydrocephalus.

Answer to Question 35
C

There is some overlap between the different types of dementia, but in this case there are clues that this is dementia with Lewy bodies (DLB) with the early development of instability, falls and hallucinations. Other features include fluctuating cognition, depression and delusions.

Treatment is usually symptomatic, but remember that neuroleptic drugs such as haloperidol will worsen Parkinsonian features, so consider using atypical antipsychotic agents such as quetiapine. There is some evidence that the dementia may respond to anticholinesterase inhibitors.

Dementia associated with Parkinson's disease tends to occur much later in the course of the disease.

Answer to Question 36
C

Parkinson's disease is typically asymmetrical at presentation. The tremor is typically a rest tremor so it is usually possible for the patient to drink (unlike benign essential tremor, where action such as drinking a cup of tea makes the tremor worse). Marked chewing movements and lip-smacking suggest drug-induced Parkinsonism and an extended neck and raised eyebrows suggest progressive supranuclear palsy; the neck is characteristically flexed in Parkinson's disease. A positive glabellar tap is common in normal older people and is falling out of favour as a diagnostic sign in younger patients too.

Emergency Medicine

Answer to Question 37
C

In the context of this clinical history, which clearly suggests a viral illness, the widespread changes to ST-segments and T-waves suggest pericarditis.

With a different history the possibility of acute inferior myocardial infarction with lateral extension would require consideration.

Answer to Question 38
C

The appearances are typical of acute anterior myocardial infarction, with gross ST-segment elevation and early Q wave formation in leads V1-4.

Answer to Question 39
D, G

The other recognised ECG criterion for thrombolysis is new left bundle branch block.

Answer to Question 40
C, E

Levels should always be measured in cases of paracetamol overdose, but if a clinically significant quantity of paracetamol seems to have been taken, start N-acetyl cysteine (NAC) whilst waiting for the results – it can be stopped if it proves to be inappropriate. Clotting, liver function, renal function and electrolytes should all be checked: the best prognostic indicator is the INR.

Intolerance to NAC is rare: most reactions to it are mild and can be overcome by slowing the rate of infusion. For patients who are truly intolerant, methionine can be given up to 12 hours after paracetamol ingestion.

Patients who are anorexic for any reason, who drink significantly (>21 units/wk for men, >14 units/wk for women) or who are on enzyme-inducing drugs are at greater risk from paracetamol overdose.

Answer to Question 41
A, D

A prolonged prothrombin time is a poor prognostic factor: there is a definite risk of acute liver failure and a need for expert toxicological and hepatological advice. Metabolic acidosis, which can be detected by arterial blood gas analysis, rising venous lactate or falling venous bicarbonate, also indicate deteriorating liver function and the need for specialist advice/transfer.

Answer to Question 42
C, I

Aminophylline is a pulmonary vasodilator and can worsen VQ mismatch. Beta-2 agonists are a recognised treatment for hyperkalaemia as they drive potassium into the cells. Patients with acute asthma are usually dry: because of high intrathoracic pressure they need a high right ventricular filling pressure to maintain cardiac output. Never use low flow oxygen in this context: hypoxia kills, hypercarbia merely intoxicates. If an acute asthmatic is hypercarbic they need ventilation. IV beta-2 agonists can be life saving in patients who are too breathless to be helped by nebulisers.

The most important investigation is arterial blood gas analysis as this will give information on carbon dioxide concentration and pH. A normal carbon dioxide level is a worrying sign – it suggests a tiring asthmatic. Hyperventilation should lower the carbon dioxide concentration.

Low dose diazepam is likely to result in your appearance in a coroner's court – sedation is contraindicated, unless the patient is mechanically ventilated. The degree of pulsus paradoxus (fall in systolic blood pressure during inspiration) does correlate with the severity of attack, but use the arterial blood gases as a guide to therapy and not repeated measurement of paradox.

Answer to Question 43
D, H

The first step in basic airway management is to open the airway. This should be done with a head-tilt chin lift, unless there is suggestion of a neck injury when a jaw-thrust manoeuvre is preferred. Material in the oropharynx should be removed under direct vision. Oropharyngeal (OPA) and nasopharyngeal (NPA) airways are useful adjuncts but do not provide a definitive airway for unconscious patients.

A quick way to size an NPA is to choose one with an external diameter similar to the patient's little finger. NPAs are contraindicated in base of skull fractures. If there is a nasal fracture, the most patent nostril should be chosen. NPAs are generally better tolerated than OPAs and can be used in patients where the laryngeal reflexes are preserved.

OPAs should be sized with the length corresponding to the distance from the angle of the patient's mouth to the angle of the jaw. Inserting OPAs can trigger vomiting and laryngospasm.

Answer to Question 44
D, F

Modern non-invasive ventilation (NIV) can provide support for patients with both type 1 and type 2 respiratory failure and is increasingly being used to support patients with conditions such as motor neurone disease, where it is mainly CO_2 clearance that is the problem. It should not be used for patients with immediate life-threatening hypoxia or ventilatory failure.

NIV should not be used in those who are comatose: it does not provide a definitive airway and the patient would be at risk of aspiration. NIV increases the risk of aspiration because raised inspiratory pressure can result in aerophagia: a nasogastric tube may be beneficial if the patient has problems with gastric distension, but this is not required in most cases.

Patients with sleep apnoea suffer from recurrent episodes of arterial desaturation. The application of continuous positive airway pressure helps to reduce these. Expiratory effort is increased as the patient is expiring against resistance, but inspiratory effort and the overall work of breathing are reduced. Functional residual capacity is increased. Common complications of NIV include claustrophobia, gastric distension and eye irritation. Continual pressure from a tight fitting mask may result in skin necrosis.

Answer to Question 45
D, G

The patient's symptoms result from his bradycardia and the pacemaker is failing to capture. The first thing to do is to check the leads. If they are connected, then the pacemaker voltage should be increased to maximum which may enable it to capture.

The threshold for pacing increases with time and should be checked at least daily. If capture occurs, arrangements should be made to reposition the pacemaker lead. If it does not, external pacing should be instituted. Cough and percussion pacing are emergency measures that occasionally work. Isoprenaline can also be effective.

Answer to Question 46
C

Tricyclic overdose can cause coma, convulsions and arrhythmias in serious cases. The single most important investigation to determine prognosis and guide therapy is a 12 lead ECG: a QRS duration >160 ms is associated with high risk of arrhythmias and the patient should be managed on a CCU / HDU. Always check for other poisons in cases of polypharmacy overdose, also check arterial blood gases for signs of hypoventilation and acidosis, but these are not the most appropriate immediate investigations in this case.

Answer to Question 47
A

The history suggests a subarachnoid haemorrhage (SAH). Urgent CT brain scan will identify more than 95% of patients with suspected subarachnoid haemorrhage if performed within 1–2 days after headache onset. Lumbar puncture is potentially dangerous in a case where there might be raised intracranial pressure and will add no extra information if brain CT shows definite evidence of extravasated blood. If CT is negative and there are no contraindications, then LP should be performed.

When the patient has stabilised, four vessel angiography will be needed to identify the source of the bleeding, which may be amenable to endovascular or surgical treatment. CT imaging is superior to MRI in acute SAH because of the speed of investigation and availability. MRI imaging becomes more useful if presentation is delayed because CT sensitivity for subarachnoid blood rapidly declines after the first few days (>4). MR angiography is without risks and reasonably sensitive (90%): it is useful for screening people at risk of intracranial

aneurysms, but less suitable for patients with subarachnoid haemorrhage.

Answer to Question 48
A

The immediate priority is to protect the heart from the effects of hyperkalaemia. This can best be done with intravenous calcium gluconate 10% 10–20 mls IV which acts instantly to 'stabilise' the cardiac membranes. The other options listed are valuable treatments for hyperkalaemia, but are not the best immediate therapy in this context because they all take time to have an effect.

Answer to Question 49
A

The commonly prescribed antibiotics clarithromycin, ciprofloxacin and metronidazole enhance the anticoagulant effect of warfarin, whereas rifampicin (a potent enzyme inducing drug) diminishes the anticoagulant effect.

Although aspirin may increase the likelihood of bleeding due to its antiplatelet and gastric irritant effects, it should not cause prolongation of the INR; other non-steroidal anti-inflammatory (NSAIDs), especially azapropazone, may cause prolongation of the INR.

Carbamazepine, primidone and phenobarbitone induce liver enzymes and therefore reduce anticoagulant effect, while valproate probably increases the INR. The effect of phenytoin is unpredictable, as both prolongation and reduction of the INR have been reported.

Unlike co-proxamol, which causes prolongation of the INR, co-dydramol has no significant effect on warfarin metabolism.

Answer to Question 50
E

She has posterior circulation signs, in particular right cerebellar signs. The immediate priority must be to exclude an acute cerebellar haemorrhage that may need surgical intervention.

Answer to Question 51
B

Troponins I and T may remain elevated for up to 3 weeks after myocardial infarction and hence are not very useful for repeat events during this period, unless a rising plasma concentration can be demonstrated.

Troponins are specific markers for cardiac muscle damage, but not specific markers of ischaemia: other conditions, e.g. myocarditis, may also produce an elevated level. A good history along with ECG changes is the only evidence-based criteria on which to base a decision on thrombolysis. Troponins are more sensitive than CK-MB in the detection of minor degrees of cardiac muscle damage and can be used as prognostic markers in the risk stratification of Acute Coronary Syndromes.

Answer to Question 52
A

The history suggests a mechanical cause and all routine investigations are normal. The negative Vidas D-dimer result makes pulmonary embolism very unlikely in the context of a low probability presentation, i.e. no risk factors and an alternative diagnosis.

Answer to Question 53
D

Although the presence of capture and fusion beats is pathognomonic of VT, they are rarely seen and their absence cannot be relied upon to rule out the diagnosis. Broad complex tachycardia in the first week after a myocardial infarction is proven to be ventricular in origin in over 90% of cases. Adenosine may induce bronchospasm and should be avoided in patients with a history of asthma. The absence of bundle branch block on a recent ECG is an unreliable indicator of the source of the tachycardia, since bundle branch block is frequently rate-related, and often resolves on termination of the dysrhythmia.

Answer to Question 54
D

Balloon tamponade is the most effective treatment for control of variceal bleeding if endoscopic therapy has failed. Even though the varices were bleeding from within the oesophagus, inflation of the gastric balloon with application of traction usually stops the bleeding by compressing the vessels as they cross the gastrooesophageal junction. Rarely, inflation of the oesophageal balloon may be required.

It is unlikely that repeat endoscopy would prevent on-going bleeding if he has already received successful sclerotherapy, unless there was doubt about the source of bleeding previously. Octreotide is less effective than terlipressin in controlling portal pressure, and therefore switching therapy is unlikely to be helpful. Although the effects of the fresh frozen plasma administered earlier will

probably have worn off, vitamin K is unlikely to help as the coagulopathy is probably due to synthetic dysfunction rather than vitamin K deficiency. Surgical transection of the oesophagus is rarely indicated, and has largely been superseded by radiological shunt insertion (e.g. TIPSS).

Answer to Question 55
D

It is likely that this patient is bleeding from oesophageal varices caused by alcohol-induced portal hypertension. Terlipressin reduces the likelihood of continued bleeding by reducing portal pressure and may be helpful prior to endoscopy, or as an adjunct to endoscopic therapy.

Intravenous omeprazole reduces the likelihood of peptic ulcer re-bleeding after endoscopic therapy, but there is no evidence to support its use as an empirical therapy before endoscopy or in the management of variceal haemorrhage. Tranexamic acid is an antifibrinolytic and has been shown to slightly reduce mortality following peptic ulcer haemorrhage in one meta-analysis, while intravenous ranitidine has no impact on outcome of upper GI bleeding from any source. Propranolol is helpful in the primary and secondary prevention of variceal haemorrhage but has no role in the acute setting.

Answer to Question 56
D

Optic atrophy suggests a diagnosis of demyelination. A clear-cut sensory level classically occurs with cord compression, and ankle weakness with saddle area sensory loss would point towards a cauda equina lesion (always examine the saddle area!). In Guillain-Barré syndrome (GBS) there are often cardiovascular abnormalities reflecting autonomic dysfunction. These can be a major problem, manifesting as extreme hypertension or hypotension, tachycardia and bradycardia, and most dramatically as sudden death. In GBS the weakness is greater distally.

Answer to Question 57
E

She has no signs of infection and is not clinically constipated. There is no history of alcohol abuse and there would often be a biochemical or haematological pointer to high alcohol intake such as abnormal liver function tests or raised MCV. Benzodiazepine withdrawal can present with acute confusion and is the most likely explanation in this case.

Answer to Question 58

C

Corticosteroids reduce the duration of a relapse, including optic neuritis, but have no effect on the disease progression or frequency of relapses. Short courses of oral or intravenous methylprednisolone have been shown to be equally effective. Avascular necrosis is a recognised side effect.

Answer to Question 59

D

DKA is associated with a high anion gap acidosis.

Answer to Question 60

E

The working diagnosis must be meningococcal meningitis and the woman must be given an appropriate antibiotic (e.g. cefotaxime 2 g) intravenously without delay. In the very old or immunocompromised it would be appropriate to add ampicillin 2 g six-hourly to cover Listeria, and aciclovir (10 mg/kg eight-hourly, with dose reduction in renal failure) should also be given if herpes simplex encephalitis is a possibility.

Answer to Question 61

A

The working diagnosis must be opioid overdose, the treatment for which is intravenous naloxone (0.4 mg), repeated up to a total dose of 2 mg depending on clinical response. The half-life of naloxone is shorter than that of opioids, hence if this man wakes up it can be anticipated that he will 're-narcose'. Repeated doses on naloxone may be required; sometime a naloxone infusion is necessary.

Answer to Question 62

E

The base excess is a figure calculated by many blood gas machines to aid interpretation of data. The principles of the calculation are as follows: predict the pH that would arise in normal blood in the presence of the pCO_2 actually measured; then calculate the amount of base that would have to be added to the blood to change the calculated pH into the pH as actually measured. This value is the base deficit or excess, in mmol/l, which quantifies the metabolic component of acid-base disturbance.

Renal failure causes metabolic acidosis with compensatory respiratory alkalosis. In this man the predicted pH (on the basis of measured pCO_2 3.2 kPa) would be alkalotic, and base would have to be removed from the blood to change this to the acidotic value actually measured (pH 7.12). This is expressed as a NEGATIVE base excess.

Answer to Question 63

D

A normal or elevated pCO_2 in an asthmatic indicates failing respiratory effort, and although this woman's oxygen saturation is not severely depressed she is in danger of decompensation and – aside from high flow oxygen, nebulised salbutamol and ipratropium, and steroids – it would be prudent to inform the ICU of her existence. The gases are not bad enough, however, to suggest that cardio-respiratory arrest is imminent.

Pneumothorax must be excluded in any asthmatic, but the presence or absence of pneumothorax can never be inferred from arterial blood gas analysis.

Answer to Question 64

C

Beta-2 agonists are pulmonary vasodilators as well as bronchodilators. Their administration can rapidly worsen the V/Q mismatch that is the cause of hypoxia in asthma and they can therefore cause reduction in arterial oxygen tension unless supplemental oxygen is given. This man should be given the highest inspired oxygen concentration that can be obtained. It would also be reasonable to mix ipratropium bromide (500 µg) with the salbutamol given in option C.

Answer to Question 65

A

The European Resuscitation Council guidelines for adult Advanced Life Support suggest that – after Basic Life Support and a precordial thump (if appropriate) – VF/VT should be treated with up to three defibrillation shocks, the first two at 200 J and the third at 360 J.

Answer to Question 66

E

Activated charcoal provides a large area for adsorption of many drugs ingested as an overdose. Examples of agents not adsorbed by activated charcoal include metals (lithium, iron), hydrocarbons and solvents, alcohols, acids and alkalis.

Infectious Diseases

Answer to Question 67
G, H

The most likely diagnosis is gas gangrene with clostridial infection. Bacteraemia complicates about 15% of patients with gas gangrene. Treatment includes emergency surgical exploration and debridement. The combination of intravenous penicillin and clindamycin is a widely used treatment once the diagnosis has been confirmed.

Further information should be obtained about the nature of this man's job. Though less likely, anthrax is also a possibility. Cases have been reported in postal workers in the USA and those who work with contaminated hides and leather. Intravenous ciprofloxacin is the recommended antibiotic, though mortality at this stage of infection is high.

Answer to Question 68
E, G

The fluid levels within cavities are due to lung abscesses. In an intravenous drug user, *Staphylococcus aureus* would be the most likely aetiological agent and was grown from this patient. *Klebsiella pneumoniae* is another common cause of lung abscess. Other bacteria are less likely causes of lung abscesses.

Answer to Question 69
C, H

The clinical picture can be explained by a diagnosis of right-sided endocarditis with secondary septic pulmonary emboli. The Gram stain shows a candidal species. Candidal endocarditis is seen in the intravenous drug using population where the organism is inadvertently introduced as a contaminant of the intravenous cocktail.

Answer to Question 70
E, I

This presentation is typical of depression. HIV encephalopathy may present with neuropsychiatric manifestations, focal neurology or dementia. Cerebral atrophy is usually present but is also common in patients with advanced HIV disease without clinical evidence of neurological involvement. MRI scans may show areas of increased signal but can also be normal. There is a substantial increase in psychiatric morbidity in patients with HIV/AIDS and acute psychiatric illness may be precipitated by a new HIV diagnosis.

Answer to Question 71
D, E

The clinical picture suggests an acute glandular fever-like viral illness. Epstein-Barr virus (EBV) and cytomegalovirus (CMV) would both need to be considered and a likely diagnosis of EBV can be quickly established by the Paul–Bunnell test. Acute CMV infection is confirmed by detection of anti-CMV IgM (not IgG). HIV seroconversion is also likely: HIV antibody is often negative early during seroconversion and the diagnosis can be established by measuring p24 antigen or detection of high level viraemia with PCR. Acute hepatitis B would need to be considered but acute hepatitis C is subclinical. Syphilis and disseminated gonorrhoea should be considered in any sexually active person presenting with fever and rash, but in this patient an acute viral infection is suggested by the reactive lymphocytosis.

Answer to Question 72
A

Primary HBV infection in susceptible hosts can either be symptomatic or asymptomatic, the latter being commoner. Most primary infections in adults are self-limiting, but 5% do not resolve and develop into persistent infection. Asymptomatic chronic HBV carriers have normal aminotransferase levels and normal or near normal liver biopsies. Patients with chronic hepatitis B have abnormal liver function tests and histological abnormalities on liver biopsy. Cirrhosis will develop in about 20% of patients with chronic hepatitis B.

Answer to Question 73
B

There are two forms of necrotising fasciitis. Type 1 is a mixed infection of anaerobes plus facultative species such as streptococci or enterobacteriacae. It is characterised by an acute, rapidly developing infection of deep fascia, marked pain, tenderness, swelling and often crepitus with bullae and necrosis of underlying skin. Type 2 is infection with group A streptococci and is characterised by acute infection often accompanied by toxic shock, rapid progression of oedema to bullae, and necrosis of subcutaneous tissue. There is no crepitus in this form of the condition.

MRI is useful in distinguishing cellulitis from necrotising fasciitis with a 100% sensitivity and 88% specificity, but wait for this test should not delay surgical exploration for a definitive diagnosis and treatment, although the prognosis is bleak.

Answer to Question 74

E

Important organisms to consider in this context are resistant gram negative rods, including pseudomonas. The only drug with such cover in this list is tazocin, but other anti-pseudomonal regimens may be suitable. Benzylpenicillin and cefuroxime cover community-acquired pneumonias but have weaker gram negative cover.

Answer to Question 75

B

VREs are an emerging problem in hospitals, where extensive glycopeptide use may select for resistant strains. Some are teicoplanin sensitive. The new agents linezolid and quinupristin with dalfopristin (Synercid) may be active. Co-trimoxazole (Septrin) is active against some highly resistant gram negative bacteria such as *Stenotrophomonas maltophilia*.

Answer to Question 76

C

MRSA is resistant to beta-lactam antibiotics. Glycopeptides such as vancomycin are commonly used. An alternative is teicoplanin. Other drugs such as gentamicin, rifampicin and doxycycline may be active.

Answer to Question 77

A

Polyoma virus BK is associated with interstitial nephritis, can cause fever and haematuria, but more commonly presents with impairment of transplant function (rising creatinine). Reduction of immunosuppression can reduce viral replication. The other viruses listed can reactivate during immunosuppression but do not cause haematuria. Cytomegalovirus (CMV) primary infection or reactivation is the most common and most feared infective complication in the early post transplant period.

Answer to Question 78

C

Aciclovir is safe in pregnancy and chickenpox is dangerous. Steroids exacerbate chickenpox. The immunosuppression of pregnancy puts the mother as well as the fetus at risk. In early pregnancy there is a risk of fetal abnormalities (about 2%). At this late stage the main

danger is that a new born child would become infected with no transfer of antibody from the mother. In that case varicella-zoster immune globulin should be given to the child, but it has no role in therapy of the mother.

Answer to Question 79

D

Pseudomonas species are very common causes of nosocomial pneumonia on the ICU. *Strep pneumoniae* is a very common cause of community-acquired pneumonia. Staphylococcal disease due to methicillin-resistant *S. aureus* (MRSA) or methicillin-susceptible *S. aureus* (MSSA) is also reasonably common. *Legionella* is usually community-acquired and can lead to ICU admission, but is now an uncommon nosocomial infection.

Answer to Question 80

B

Erythema multiforme is a common complication of genital herpes infection. The target-like lesions appear either as the genital lesion is evolving or soon after. Attacks can be controlled with continuous oral aciclovir to prevent HSV reactivation, but aciclovir has no effect on the erythema multiforme during an acute attack.

Answer to Question 81

D

Sexually transmitted infections (STI) are unlikely with this history. Toxic shock syndrome is associated with retained tampons and can present with fevers, hypotension and rash. Unless diagnosed early patients may deteriorate rapidly and fatalities have been reported. Removal of the foreign body should be accompanied by antibiotic therapy regardless of the risk for STI.

Answer to Question 82

D

Patients often report as allergies side effects of a drug that are not related to allergic phenomenon. These commonly include nausea, diarrhoea and headache. If a patient reports a drug allergy you should always determine what the allergy was, how severe it was, and who diagnosed and/or documented it. Erythromycin is well known to cause nausea and gastrointestinal symptoms as a side effect.

Clinical manifestations of drug reactions	Onset
Anaphylaxis, urticaria	0–24 hours
Haemolytic anaemia, neutropenia, thrombocytopenia	>72 hours

Drug fever, serum sickness	7–14 days
Contact dermatitis	Variable
Rash, fixed drug reactions	>7–14 days

Answer to Question 83
D

The combination of long history, focal signs, very high protein, low glucose and a lymphocytic CSF make a diagnosis of tuberculous meningitis the most likely. The diagnosis of neurosyphilis cannot be made without a positive serum specific treponemal antibody (TPHA); the positive VDRL is a biological false positive.

Answer to Question 84
D

Penicillin allergy is reported after 0.7–4% of courses of the drug, with anaphylaxis reported following 1/32 000 to 1/100 000 courses.

Standard treatment of severe community-acquired pneumonia would involve parenteral administration of a second or third-generation cephalosporin (e.g. cefotaxime) and a macrolide (e.g. erythromycin). Patients with penicillin allergy often tolerate cephalosporins, but there is a 5–10% chance of cross-reactivity. If the previous reaction to penicillin were simply a rash you should not be dissuaded from giving a cephalosporin if there is good indication, and option A would be appropriate in this case. However, with a history of anaphylactic reaction this would clearly NOT be the correct treatment in this case and high dose intravenous erythromycin would be the treatment to use.

Answer to Question 85
C

Infective endocarditis is the only diagnosis that would explain all of the symptoms and investigative findings. Vertebral osteomyelitis/discitis and stroke are both recognised complications of infective endocarditis and either can be the presenting feature of the disease.

Answer to Question 86
C

The British Thoracic Society has published guidelines for assessment and management of adult community-acquired pneumonia. Adverse prognostic features include:
• Pre-existing factors: age > 50 years; co-existing disease
• Core clinical adverse prognostic features (CURB criteria): confusional state; urea > 7 mmol/l; respiratory rate > 30/min; systolic BP < 90 mmHg and/or diastolic BP < 60 mmHg.
• Additional features: hypoxaemia, SaO_2 < 92% or PaO_2 < 8 kPa; bilateral/multi-lobe disease.

Patients with two or more core features are at high risk of death and should be managed as severe pneumonia in hospital.

Answer to Question 87
A

The persistence of fever, timing and description of the lesions fits best with disseminated yeast infection, most likely *Candida* species. The diagnosis can usually be made on blood cultures, but the organisms can also be seen in the lesions on biopsy. Do not forget to look in the fundi in such cases. The presentation is too early for graft versus host disease.

Answer to Question 88
E

The presentation with fever, diarrhoea, shock and a macular rash are characteristic of staphylococcal toxic shock syndrome due to focal infection with a toxin-producing strain of *S. aureus*. Confusion, breathlessness (due to metabolic acidosis) and oliguria are commonly present. The toxin acts as a superantigen bypassing the normal antigen-restricted pathway of T-cell activation and leading to widespread cytokine release shock and organ failure. Approximately 50% of cases occur in young women due to vaginal infection with *S. aureus* at the time of menstruation. A retained vaginal tampon increases the risk and should be looked for in this type of presentation. A similar syndrome may also be seen with toxin producing streptococci.

Answer to Question 89
C

Tetanus and strychnine poisoning both produce muscle spasm that may lead to respiratory failure, but they do not cause muscle weakness. Rabies produces a uniformly fatal encephalitis characterised by pharyngeal spasm triggered by water. Diphtheria presents with a pharyngitis and a membrane over the tonsils: the toxin may cause myocarditis and neurotoxicity with palatal paralysis and cranial nerve palsies. Botulism typically produces a descending paralysis which starts with diplopia or blurred vision (due to difficulty with accommodation) and progresses to weakness of the neck, arms and respiratory muscles.

Answer to Question 90

C

Pneumococcus remains the commonest cause of community-acquired pneumonia. In giving empirical treatment you would want to cover for the possibility of Legionella and other atypicals (by giving clarithromycin or erythromycin), but these would be a less likely cause of this man's illness.

Answer to Question 91

D

The undetectable HIV viral load implies that the patient is receiving therapy. The blood tests point to a partially compensated metabolic acidosis with abnormal liver function tests. This syndrome is seen with nucleoside reverse transcriptase inhibitors (AZT group of drugs) and is thought to result from inhibition of mitochondrial DNA. In addition to lactic acidosis, most patients have fatty infiltration of the liver with a cholestatic pattern of liver enzymes. The initial clinical presentation is often non-specific with vague abdominal pain and bloating. Alternative diagnostic possibilities include bacterial sepsis and poisoning from salicylate or methanol, but there is nothing else to suggest these in this case.

Lactic acidosis is one of the most feared adverse effects of anti-HIV therapy and may be fatal if not recognised promptly. Most patients gradually improve after withdrawal of anti-retroviral therapy, in severe cases haemofiltration may be required to control acidosis.

Dermatology

Answer to Question 92

A

Rosacea causes erythematous papules and scattered pustules on the convex surfaces of the face, including the forehead as shown here. Telangiectasiae are a common feature. By contrast with acne, comedones are absent. There is no rash on the body.

Answer to Question 93

A, B

Although many of the diagnoses listed above can affect the hands, the commonest diagnoses in this setting would be an irritant hand dermatitis or a contact allergic der-

matitis. Possible precipitants for the latter could include rubber (including latex), hair-dye and nickel. It would be important to undertake patch testing to a wide range of potential contact allergens in order to identify the precipitant and advise on her future career.

Answer to Question 94

B, I

This is a typical case of erythema nodosum, but insect bites can give a similar picture, as can nodular vasculitis, which is much rarer. Erythema nodosum can be caused by a variety of infections (streptococci, tuberculosis, yersinia, chlamydia, Epstein-Barr virus, *Trichophyton*, coccidiomycosis), drugs (sulphonamides, oral contraceptives), as well as other conditions such as sarcoidosis, Crohn's disease, ulcerative colitis, Behçet's disease and malignancy.

Answer to Question 95

B

Polymorphic light eruption is a common photosensitivity disorder that particularly affects young women. The skin shows 'hardening', whereby areas frequently exposed to the sun, such as the face and hands, may not be affected whilst newly exposed sites are most severely affected. The rash often develops after a few days of sun exposure and is most severe at the beginning of the summer.

Systemic lupus erythematosus is a photoaggravated disorder in which the face is usually affected. Photoallergic contact dermatitis can occur due to sunscreen allergy, but a rash would appear at all sites where sunscreen had been applied and subsequently exposed to the sun. Scabies is not photoaggavated. Patients with xeroderma pigmentosum describe easy burning after minimal sun exposure and subsequently develop freckling, chronic solar damage and skin tumours.

Answer to Question 96

A

Rosacea often presents with easy facial flushing before the onset of a pustular rash. Rosacea is often mistaken for acne, but comedones are the clinical hallmark of acne and are absent in rosacea.

Carcinoid syndrome often presents with flushing but is not associated with a pustular rash. SLE can cause erythema of the cheeks but pustules are not seen. Allergic contact dermatitis would most commonly present with a scaly, eczematous rash.

Answer to Question 97

E

Allergic contact dermatitis is a type 4 (delayed) hypersensitivity reaction and is diagnosed by patch testing. Nickel is one of the commonest causes, with an increased frequency in women, probably due to increased exposure to nickel-containing jewellery, particularly through earrings for pierced ears. Men with nickel allergy are more likely to have an occupational cause. Atopic patients are thought to be less prone to developing allergic contact dermatitis (other than to medicaments). Low carat gold often contains significant amounts of nickel. This can be detected by the nickel spot test: dimethylglyoxime rubbed against a metal will turn pink in the presence of nickel.

Answer to Question 98

C

Irritant hand dermatitis classically causes dermatitis in the finger webs, beneath rings and over the dorsum of the hands. It can be caused acutely by contact with strong alkalis or acids, but is usually a chronic problem caused by repeated exposure to detergents and wet work. Atopic patients are more prone to develop irritant dermatitis.

Patch tests demonstrate type IV allergic reactions and are used to diagnose allergic contact dermatitis: they are negative in an irritant dermatitis. Histology is similar in allergic and irritant dermatitis hence the diagnosis of an irritant contact dermatitis is based on the history, clinical signs and negative patch tests. The treatment of irritant and allergic dermatitis is similar and involves avoidance of irritants/allergens, use of soap substitutes, regular emollients and topical steroids.

Answer to Question 99

A

The Koebner phenomenon is the localization of cutaneous disease to sites of trauma and is shown by several disorders including psoriasis, lichen planus, viral warts and vitiligo.

Nail involvement in psoriasis is common and characterized by the presence of 'thimble pitting', onycholysis (separation of the nail from the nail bed) and subungual hyperkeratosis. Chronic plaque psoriasis localising to the extensor surfaces is by far the commonest form. Widespread pustules within lesions or on erythematous skin should raise the possibility of generalized pustular psoriasis, which is a rare but serious complication with a significant mortality. Although pruritus can be feature of psoriasis, it is rarely intense.

Haematology

Answer to Question 100

D

Acute leukaemia, myeloma and lymphoma can all present with neck swelling, but the appearances of myeloma cells on the aspirate are characteristic. The plasma cells do not look granular and have too much cytoplasm for acute leukaemia, and lymphoma cells tend to have rather less cytoplasm and irregular nuclei.

Answer to Question 101

A

The CT scan shows bilateral psoas abscesses, caused in this case by methicillin-resistant *Staphylococcus aureus* (MRSA), presumed related to a previous Hickman line infection.

Answer to Question 102

B

Factitious purpura occurs in a linear fashion over parts of the body that are easily scratched by the patient.

As a general rule, purpura affect the lower legs rather than the thighs. The normal platelet count and clotting make a primary haematological problem unlikely, and the appearances are not at all typical of either Henoch-Schönlein purpura or purpura fulminans.

Answer to Question 103

C

The combination of fever, neurological impairment and mild renal impairment is typical of thrombotic thrombocytopenic purpura, confirmed in this case by the finding of severe thrombocytopenia and microangiopathic appearances on the blood film.

Answer to Question 104

D

Patients who require recurrent venesection typically become iron deficient. The iron should not be replaced: if it is, then haemoglobin will rise above normal levels.

Answer to Question 105

E

Patients without a spleen are prone to Overwhelming Post Splenectomy Infection (OPSI) that involves encapsulated organisms including pneumococcus, meningococcus and *Haemophilus influenzae*. They are also prone to severe falciparum malarial infection and *Capnocytophagia canimorsus* bacterium. The spleen is necessary for filtering, phagocytosis and production of antibodies required for opsonisation of these bacteria and protozoa. Lifelong penicillin is recommended but compliance is very poor, hence some physicians recommend 3 g amoxicillin to be taken at onset of febrile illness, with erythromycin as an alternative in those who are penicillin sensitive.

Answer to Question 106

C

The most appropriate treatment for this man with symptomatic ITP is intravenous immunoglobulin. Oral steroids will work in 60–70% of cases but take about 2–3 days before an effect is noted. It is possible to give massive platelet transfusions to swamp the antibody, but the hazards of blood transfusions need to be borne in mind. In ITP the thrombopoietin levels are high and no commercially available thrombopoietin is in routine use.

Answer to Question 107

D

Haemostasis and thrombosis are finely regulated processes that depend on the level and configuration of prothrombotic proteins and natural anticoagulants. They can either be inherited or acquired. The inherited thrombophilias are:

- Activated Protein C (APC) resistance due to an abnormal Factor VL, i.e. Factor V Leiden
- Protein C deficiency
- Protein S deficiency
- Antithrombin III deficiency

Inherited hyperhomocysteinaemia is also associated with arterial and venous thrombosis.

The lupus anticoagulant is an acquired anticoagulant that prolongs phospholipid dependent tests *in vitro* but predisposes to thrombosis in patients. In up to 50% of cases of venous thrombosis it is possible to demonstrate an inherited abnormality of coagulation.

Factor VIII deficiency is an X-linked predisposition to bleeding called haemophilia A.

Answer to Question 108

D

Ferritin is an acute phase reactant, hence a normal value does not exclude iron deficiency anaemia. A low ferritin would be a useful result, strongly supporting the diagnosis of iron deficiency.

Anaemia of chronic disorders is a feature of rheumatoid arthritis, most marked in the acute phase of the illness. Felty's syndrome is very uncommon.

The differential diagnosis of her anaemia is wide. Appropriate tests would include: B12, folate, iron, total iron binding capacity, ferritin; inflammatory markers (C-reactive protein); thyroid function; rheumatoid factor; immunoglobulins (could this be myeloma?); liver, renal and bone function tests; chest radiograph.

Answer to Question 109

E

This is a typical presentation of acute chest syndrome, which is one of the commonest causes of death in adults with sickle cell disease. Pulmonary embolism and pneumonia cannot be excluded, but are less likely diagnoses.

Key aspects of management are:
- Give high flow oxygen via reservoir bag
- Rapid intravenous infusion of 1 litre of 0.9% saline
- Start intravenous antibiotics, e.g. ampicillin 500 mg qds
- Intravenous opioid for pain, e.g. diamorphine 5 mg, with antiemetic
- Prophylaxis against venous thromboembolism, e.g. enoxaparin 20 mg SC od
- Call for specialist advice if the patient deteriorates or does not improve rapidly
- Exchange transfusion may be indicated if the patient becomes hypoxic

Answer to Question 110

A

Thrombocytosis is much more commonly a secondary phenomenon than part of a primary malignant process. Blood loss results in increased marrow activity and hence a raised platelet count. Treatment of the underlying cause will serve to bring the platelet count down gradually.

Answer to Question 111

D

The diagnosis is gestational thrombocytopenia, which is seen in 1–4% of pregnancies and suggested in this case by the history of a similar picture in a previous pregnancy. Idiopathic thrombocytopenic purpura (ITP) and haemolysis/elevated liver enzyme/low platelets (HELLP) syndrome are unlikely in someone who is asymptomatic, in particular in the absence of petechiae/

purpura. HIV-infection can cause thrombocytopenia, but absence of risk factors make it unlikely here. The baby should have the platelet count checked at birth and a week later.

Answer to Question 112

E

Hodgkin's disease (HD) and non-Hodgkin's lymphoma can both present with isolated cervical lymphadenopathy, but this is more commonly seen in HD in this age group. The node(s) are classically painless and non-tender. The patient is often otherwise well, but may have 'B' symptoms (weight loss, fevers and night sweats).

Oncology

Answer to Question 113

A

Basal cell carcinomas start as painless translucent pearly nodules with telangiectasia on sun-exposed skin. They ulcerate as they enlarge and develop a rolled shiny edge, progressing slowly over months to years. They are very common on the face, especially the nose, nasolabial fold and inner canthus.

Answer to Question 114

E

The chest radiograph (Figure 17) shows diffuse interstitial fibrosis, most prominent in the lower zones, typical of bleomycin toxicity.

Answer to Question 115

B, E

It is not known whether radiotherapy followed by surgical resection (option B) or surgical resection followed by radiotherapy depending on findings at operation (option E) produces the best outcome. A Medical Research Council (MRC) trial (to which many hospitals in the UK are recruiting patients) is currently comparing these two treatments.

If locally advanced disease (spread to local lymph nodes, Dukes' Grade C) is found at surgery, then adjuvant chemotherapy improves median and symptom-free survival. The mainstay of colorectal chemotherapy is 5-fluorouracil/folinic acid combination.

Answer to Question 116

H, I

Meticulous examination of the scalp and skin of the head and neck for a primary tumour, together with thorough ENT examination, are essential, but if these do not reveal a primary tumour, then cervical cancer or lung cancer are the most likely sites for a primary. Investigation should include colposcopy and Papanicolou smear test and chest radiography. If these do not reveal a primary, then barium swallow or upper gastrointestinal endoscopy with oesophageal biopsies would be appropriate to look for oesophageal carcinoma.

Patients presenting with high cervical lymphadenopathy containing squamous cell carcinoma may have occult tumours of the nasopharynx, oropharynx or hypopharynx. In such cases radical neck dissection followed by extended field radiotherapy that includes these possible primary sites may yield five-year survival rates of 30%. However, lower cervical lymphadenopathy – as in this case – has a much worse prognosis and should not be treated in this way.

Answer to Question 117

H, I

For malignant mesothelioma, the prognostic scoring systems of the Cancer and Leukaemia Group B (CALGB) and European Organisation for Research and Treatment of Cancer (EORTC) are the most useful. They rate performance status, age, histological subtype, weight loss and haematological parameters as the most useful prognostic factors.

Answer to Question 118

C

Radiation-induced sarcomas are very rare: they occur from 7 years onwards after radiotherapy.

Answer to Question 119

C

The risk of developing breast cancer in the general population is approximately 8%. Patients with a strong family history of breast cancer are at a higher risk, and this is especially true if one of the family members was young at the time of their presentation. The overall relative risk of breast cancer in a woman with an affected first-degree relative is 1.7. Premenopausal onset in a first-degree relative is associated with a three-fold increase in relative risk, whereas postmenopausal diagnosis increases the relative risk by only 1.5. No increase in risk has been demonstrated when only a second-degree relative (aunt, cousin, grandmother) is affected. The risk in this patient is approximately three-fold higher than the general population.

Some inherited breast cancers are associated with a gene called BRCA1 on chromosome 17. This gene is mutated in some families with early-onset breast cancer and ovarian cancer, and about 85% of women with BRCA1 gene mutations will develop breast cancer in their lifetime. Other genes have been identified that are associated with increased risk of breast and other cancers, including BRCA2, ataxia-telangiectasia mutation, p53.

Genetic testing is available for women at high risk of breast cancer, but this is controversial as problems associated with management of those with identified mutations, their insurability, and potential social conflicts can be anticipated.

Answer to Question 120

C

The patient has carcinoid syndrome due to an underlying carcinoid tumour. These tumours may contain and secrete a number of biologically active substances, including adrenocorticotrophic hormone (ACTH), gastrin, beta-somatostatin, insulin, motilin, growth hormone, gastrin-releasing peptide, serotonin, calcitonin, neurotensin, beta-melanocyte stimulating hormone, tachykinins (substance P, substance K, neuropeptide K), glucagon, pancreatic polypeptide (PP), vasoactive intestinal peptide (VIP) and prostaglandins. These substances may not be released in sufficient amounts to cause symptoms. 5-hydroxyindoleacetic acid is the metabolic product excreted in urine from the metabolism of serotonin.

Ectopic ACTH production with Cushing's syndrome is increasingly seen with foregut carcinoids and in some studies these tumours have been the most common cause of the ectopic ACTH syndrome. Acromegaly due to release of growth hormone-releasing factors can also occur with carcinoids.

Answer to Question 121

E

In good performance status patients with limited metastatic disease, nephrectomy plus immunotherapy offers longer survival than immunotherapy alone.

Answer to Question 122

B

The overall 5-year survival of patients with ovarian cancer that extends beyond the ovaries is 40%. How-ever, some patients who are able to undergo complete or nearly complete initial cytoreductive surgery can be cured with combination chemotherapy, which presumably eradicates residual subclinical disease that is invariably present despite apparently complete resection. Effective drugs include taxol, cisplatin, cyclophosphamide, hexamethylmelamine, and doxorubicin. Paclitaxel plus cisplatin is the standard regimen.

Answer to Question 123

B

It is likely that he has a right apical carcinoma of the lung causing a Horner's syndrome (ipsilateral ptosis, meiosis and anhydrosis). Small cell lung cancer generally arises centrally as opposed to the more peripheral lesions of non-small cell lung cancer. Squamous cell carcinoma accounts for about 30% of all lung cancers and arises most frequently in proximal segmental bronchi. Most of adenocarcinomas of the lung are peripheral in origin. The tumour in this case is on the right and not the left.

Answer to Question 124

D

Almost all forms of paraneoplastic syndromes with lung cancer are commoner with small cell lung cancer, except clubbing, hypercalcaemia and hypertrophic pulmonary osteoarthropathy (HPOA) which are more frequent with squamous cell tumours.

Answer to Question 125

B

This is a low risk melanoma. Excision margins greater than 1–2 cm have no advantage and the role of adjuvant immunotherapy is debatable, even in high risk patients, although it may prolong disease-free survival. Sentinel node biopsy is in clinical trial for thicker melanomas.

Answer to Question 126

A

A normal person excretes up to 150 mg of protein per day, which is chiefly Tamm-Horsfall mucoprotein. Dipsticks can detect as little as 50 mg protein per litre, but a false negative result occurs with immunoglobulins, which are positively charged.

Answer to Question 127

B

Peripheral neuropathy, the most frequent neurotoxicity of chemotherapy, is commonly seen with vinca alkaloids, taxanes and platinum derivatives. It usually presents as symmetrical sensory loss that may progress to worsening paraesthesia, loss of tendon reflexes and eventually motor weakness due to axonal degeneration. Features usually slowly improve over several months following cessation of chemotherapy, although residual deficits may persist indefinitely.

Cardiology

Answer to Question 128
D

The ECG (Figure 18) shows a short PR interval and δ waves, diagnostic of the Wolff-Parkinson-White syndrome.

Answer to Question 129
D

The ECG (Figure 19) shows ST segment elevation in leads V1-4(5) consistent with acute anterior myocardial infarction, and there are ventricular ectopics. There is no significant ST segment elevation in leads I, AVL or V6, as would be expected with lateral extension, and there are no features of posterior extension.

Answer to Question 130
C, I

Cardiac complications of Marfan's are relatively common. Usually they are related to aortic involvement, but Marfan's is associated with mitral valve prolapse and regurgitation, left ventricular dilatation and cardiac failure, pulmonary artery dilatation and regurgitation of the pulmonary valve.

Answer to Question 131
F, G

The patient has a non-ST-segment elevation myocardial infarction (NSTEMI) and has a high risk of further adverse cardiac events. The mainstay of initial treatment is aggressive anti-platelet therapy: aspirin with the addition of clopidogrel, and consideration of an infusion of Glycoprotein IIb/IIa receptor blocker (blocks the platelet receptor). A therapeutic dose of low molecular weight heparin should be commenced, and early angiography and percutaneous coronary intervention should be considered. Thrombolysis has not been shown to benefit patients with NSTEMI.

Answer to Question 132
G, H

All of the conditions listed, excepting hypothyroidism, might explain hypertension, but all other than essential hypertension and 'white coat' hypertension are rare (together accounting for less than 5% of cases). Although a secondary cause of hypertension is very unlikely it would be important to look for clues in history and examination that might suggest renovascular disease (ischaemic heart disease, transient ischmaemic attack (TIA)/stroke, peripheral vascular disease), renal disease (previous nephritis, results of urine testing for e.g. insurance/employment medicals). Episodes of palpitations, sweating or headache may suggest phaeochromocytoma, but a less exotic cause such as anxiety would be a much more likely explanation. The serum potassium concentration is just below the lower limit of normal, but primary hyperaldosteronism (Conn's syndrome) remains exceedingly unlikely. In the case of an obese man it is also important to note that the blood pressure reading may be falsely elevated as a result of inadequate blood pressure cuff size, and it would be important to ensure that readings were taken with appropriate equipment.

Answer to Question 133
B

Exercise testing has long been an established method for identifying patients with underlying coronary disease. Apart from changes in the ST segments, other features associated with underlying disease and adverse prognosis are ventricular arrhythmias, inadequate blood pressure response, inadequate heart rate response and angina.

Answer to Question 134
C

Patients with heart failure are considered for cardiac transplantation when significant symptoms persist despite maximal medical therapy. Due to the shortage of donors clinical guidelines have been established highlighting patients most suitable for transplantation. Significant impairment of renal function is generally considered to be a contraindication, assuming this is not reversible.

Patients with prior history of cancer may be considered if there is no evidence recurrence (>5 years on from diagnosis of cancer).

Answer to Question 135
B

Beta-blockers have prognostic and symptomatic benefit in heart failure. In the UK only carvedilol and bisoprolol are licensed for this use. Digoxin can improve symptoms in severe heart failure. Whilst it may well slow resting heart rate in atrial fibrillation it has less benefit on exercise related increases in rate. This patient has permanent atrial fibrillation and DC cardioversion will not, by definition, restore sinus rhythm.

Answer to Question 136
B

Unless it is definitely known that a patient has a tendency to retain carbon dioxide, all patients with severe breathlessness should be given high flow oxygen via a reservoir bag once it has been established that their airway is clear. After the patient has been started on high flow oxygen, give furosemide 40–80 mg IV and diamorphine 2.5–5 mg IV. If matters do not improve consider isosorbide dinitrate 2–10 mg/hr IV. If matters worsen, then call the Intensive Care Unit (ICU) sooner rather than later (assuming that the man's condition prior to this acute presentation means that this is appropriate). Concurrently try to establish a cause for the acute deterioration: has he had a myocardial infarction? If so, would he benefit from thrombolysis?

Answer to Question 137
D

Anterior myocardial infarction is typically associated with an apical ventricular septal defect (VSD), whilst inferior myocardial infarction is more commonly associated with a basal VSD or posterior papillary muscle rupture. After confirmation of diagnosis by echocardiography or right heart catheter, which reveals a step up in oxygenation at ventricular level, urgent referral to a surgical centre is required, the outlook without surgical repair being extremely poor. Anterior myocardial infarction associated with an apical VSD carries a better surgical outlook than inferior myocardial infarction associated with basal VSD.

Answer to Question 138
C

The top priority is to achieve myocardial reperfusion. The presence of chest pain and ST segment elevation on ECG indicate that thrombolysis is needed immediately, notwithstanding the presence of Q waves.

Answer to Question 139
D

Drug treatment to lower serum cholesterol should be based on a person's risk of an ischaemic heart disease (IHD) event rather than initial cholesterol level. Any person who has had a myocardial infarction has about a 10% chance (without treatment) of dying from ischaemic heart disease in the following year, and about a 5% chance of IHD death in each year thereafter. All such people (in the absence of contraindications to the specific drugs) qualify for HMG-coenzyme A reductase inhibitor therapy (statins) regardless of their cholesterol level. There is a constant proportional relationship between serum cholesterol and disease risk, so any reduction in cholesterol level from any starting point leads to the same proportional reduction in IHD risk. Those people with the highest absolute starting risk (namely those with preexisting IHD, such as this man who has had an AMI) stand to benefit the most. Non-pharmacological means of serum cholesterol reduction are far less effective, and whilst important are inadequate as sole treatment in this patient.

Answer to Question 140
A

The combination of a young patient and a 'flu-like illness makes acute viral pericarditis the most likely diagnosis in this case. The chest pain of pericarditis can be indistinguishable from that of myocardial infarction, excepting that sitting forward often eases it. The key physical sign to elicit would be a pericardial rub, and the key initial investigation would be the ECG, looking for widespread ST segment elevation, concave upwards.

Answer to Question 141
B

A normal lung perfusion scan has a specificity of around 98% for pulmonary embolism (PE), whilst specificity for CT is usually quoted at around 85% because small peripheral clots may be missed. CT scanning may, however, reveal an alternative explanation for a patient's symptoms. Although a negative D-dimer test is helpful in the context of a low index of clinical suspicion, some studies have indicated a false negative rate as high as 20% for patients with high clinical probability and most algorithms would not sanction the use of D-dimer testing at all in patients with high clinical probability. Neither normal chest radiograph, normal arterial blood gases, nor the absence of deep venous thrombosis (DVT) can be used in isolation to rule out pulmonary embolism, although they may all be helpful as part of an algorithm for the management of patients with breathlessness or pleuritic chest pain of uncertain cause.

Answer to Question 142
C

Breathlessness is the commonest symptom of pulmonary embolism (PE), and syncope is a less common (and often poorly recognised) presenting symptom. The patient is hypoxic with an oxygen saturation of only 92% on 40% oxygen, and he has non-specific but recognised ECG changes of PE. His recent varicose vein surgery is a risk factor.

Acute myocardial infarction rarely presents with syncope with no ECG changes, and ongoing hypoxia would not be explained with a 'normal' chest radiograph. Chronic obstructive pulmonary disease (COPD) is also unlikely as the cause of syncope with little evidence of severe airways obstruction.

Respiratory Medicine

Answer to Question 143
A

The radiograph (Figure 20) shows a left hilar mass, which proved to be a large-cell carcinoma.

Answer to Question 144
B

There is opacification obscuring the right heart border due to right middle lobe collapse.

Answer to Question 145
A, D

The most likely diagnosis to explain gradually worsening breathlessness with regular sputum production is bron-

chiectasis. This could arise as a consequence of childhood infection (measles, pneumonia, pertussis), cystic fibrosis, alpha 1 antitrypsin deficiency or hypogammaglobulinaemia (which would be suggested by recurrent pneumonia or sinusitis).

Answer to Question 146
C, H

The spirometry effectively rules out obstructive lung disease/asthma. Hypoxia excludes hyperventilation and anaemia as primary causes. The differential diagnosis lies between diffuse parenchymal lung disease and a problem with the pulmonary vasculature.

In diffuse parenchymal lung disease the patient may have a dry cough, but there may be no specific features. It will be important to ask about systemic / iatrogenic disorders associated with lung disease, and specific employment history / recreational interests may also be relevant. Note that the chest radiograph can appear entirely normal in patients with diffuse parenchymal lung disease. Regarding diseases of the pulmonary vasculature, a small number of patients with pulmonary embolism present with breathlessness alone, but primary pulmonary hypertension needs careful consideration in this case.

Answer to Question 147
A, I

Drug-induced pulmonary eosinophilia is the most common type of pulmonary eosinophilia seen in the western world. Drugs that can be responsible include ampicillin, aspirin, captopril, bleomycin, carbamazepine, dapsone, ethambutol, gold, methotrexate, penicillin, penicillamine, sulphonamides (including sulfasalazine), tamoxifen and tetracycline.

Answer to Question 148
C

Normal spirometry excludes chronic obstructive pulmonary disease. Raynaud's syndrome with telangiectasia and radiological appearances suggestive of pulmonary hypertension with impaired gas transfer are most likely due to a vasculitic process in pulmonary circulation associated with an autoimmune rheumatic disorder.

Answer to Question 149
C

Polymyositis and dermatomyositis are inflammatory conditions involving the muscle and skin. Patients often complain of proximal muscle weakness and of pain in the small joints of the fingers. They may have ragged cuticles and haemorrhages at the finger nail folds. Interstitial lung disease can occur. Underlying malignancy (lungs, ovaries, breasts and stomach) is present in 5–8% of cases.

Answer to Question 150

B

The patient has both lung and kidney involvement typical of a 'pulmonary renal syndrome'. Goodpasture described the association of pulmonary haemorrhage with renal failure (Goodpasture's syndrome) in 1919, and the 'classic' cause of this, where the condition is due to the presence of circulating anti-glomerular basement membrane antibodies (anti-GBM antibodies) is termed Goodpasture's disease (although this wasn't the cause of the cases he described). Other causes of pulmonary haemorrhage and renal failure include Wegener's granulomatosis, microscopic polyangiitis and systemic lupus erythematous (SLE).

Answer to Question 151

D

The combination of bilateral hilar lymphadenopathy and erythema nodosum is diagnostic of sarcoidosis. This is usually self-limiting. She should however be followed up in clinic with full lung function tests including transfer factor and lung volumes. Serum angiotensin-converting enzyme (ACE) level and lung function can be used to monitor disease. Worsening disease should be treated with prednisolone.

Answer to Question 152

A

Infected pleural effusions should be drained. In this clinical context a pleural effusion should be drained if the pH < 7.2, Gram stain shows organisms, the fluid is frankly purulent, or if clinical improvement is slow despite antibiotics.

Answer to Question 153

D

Restrictive lung disorders are characterised by reduced FEV1 & FVC, FEV1/FVC > 70%, reduced TLC & RV and reduced TLCO.

Obstructive disorders are characterised by reduced FEV1 & FVC, FEV1/FVC < 70%, raised TLC & RV (gas trapping) and reduced TLCO (emphysema) or normal or raised TLCO (non-smoking asthmatics).

Mixed disorders may have reduced FEV1 & FVC, FEV1/FVC < 70% and raised TLC & RV, reduced, normal or raised TLCO depending on whether the obstructive disorder is due to emphysema or asthma.

Answer to Question 154

D

Reduced FEV1 and FVC with normal FEV1 ratio is compatible with restrictive defect.

Answer to Question 155

E

The first investigation should be diagnostic aspiration of pleural fluid for biochemical, microbiological and cytological analysis. Light's criteria can be used to distinguish transudates from exudates: in exudates at least one of the following three criteria are met—pleural fluid protein concentration greater than 50% of that in plasma; pleural fluid LDH greater than 60% of that in plasma; pleural fluid LDH more that two thirds the upper limit of normal in plasma. Transudative pleural effusions are most commonly due to congestive cardiac failure but are sometimes associated with hypoproteinaemic states such as cirrhosis or nephrotic syndrome. Most other causes of pleural effusion are exudative.

Answer to Question 156

D

Although obtructive sleep apnoea can cause chronic respiratory failure, it is unusual to have chronic type 2 respiratory failure except in combination with some other cardiopulmonary illness. This blood gas would be most compatible with a patient with severe chronic obstructive pulmonary disease and chronic type 2 respiratory failure with an acute exacerbation.

Answer to Question 157

D

Initially the history might suggest a number of diagnoses, including cardiac tamponade, massive pulmonary embolism, haemothorax or aortic dissection, but the respiratory examination findings indicate that he almost certainly has sustained a spontaneous pneumothorax that has now developed into a tension pneumothorax. The scenario indicates that the man is about to suffer a cardiorespiratory arrest: there is no time to arrange for portable chest radiograph before attempting to reduce the pressure in the right hemithorax with the insertion of a large bore needle. If the diagnosis is correct, insertion may be accompanied by a loud 'hiss'. Positive pressure ventilation is relatively contraindicated in this situation, and will probably not be required once the lung has re-inflated.

Gastroenterology and Hepatology

Answer to Question 158
E

The CT scan (Figure 22) shows multiple hepatic cysts and ascites, the uniformly grey area seen anterior to the cystic liver. Both kidneys had been surgically removed several years ago and are not visible on the scan!

Many patients with autosomal dominant polycystic kidney disease have liver cysts, which can sometimes cause massive hepatomegally but rarely cause liver dysfunction.

Answer to Question 159
C

The appearances are typical of a benign oesophageal stricture caused by oesophageal reflux.

Answer to Question 160
F, I

The three commonest causes of acute liver failure are paracetamol overdose, non-A non-B non-C viral hepatitis (cryptogenic) and drug-induced. Has he taken an overdose, and has he been exposed to any new drug in the last two weeks, particularly a non-steroidal anti-inflammatory agent? Is he at risk of exposure to hepatitis B?

In cases of paracetamol overdose remember that N-acetylcysteine improves prognosis, even in patients who present more than 16 hr afterwards. On day 2 (24–48 hours) after a paracetamol overdose the indications for referral to a specialist centre for consideration of transplantation are arterial pH < 7.3, INR > 3, encephalopathy, creatinine >200 µmol/l or hypoglycaemia.

Answer to Question 161
D, H

The presentation with gastrointestinal symptoms occurs on a background suggesting a systemic component to the illness, hence the most likely diagnoses are an inflammatory mass associated with Crohn's disease or an appendix

abscess. In an older patient caecal carcinoma would be a more likely explanation.

Aside from assessment of cardiovascular status (is resuscitation required?) and for the presence of peritonism (which would suggest a perforated viscus and the need for laparotomy), examine carefully for signs that would support a diagnosis of Crohn's disease. These include clubbing, aphthous ulceration, perianal skin tags/ulceration/fistulae and (less commonly) seronegative arthritis, sacroiliitis, iritis and skin rashes (erythema nodosum, pyoderma gangrenosum).

Answer to Question 162
C, D

Gallstones (30–50%) and alcohol (10–40%) account for the most cases of acute pancreatitis. Less common causes include drugs (e.g. azathioprine, sulphasalazine, furosemide), toxins, trauma (blunt trauma to the abdomen as well as iatrogenic trauma, e.g. postoperative and ERCP), hypertriglyceridemia, hypercalcaemia, infections (e.g. mumps, Coxsackie, cytomegalovirus), congenital anomalies (pancreas divisum, choledochocele), ampullary or pancreatic tumors, vascular abnormalities (atherosclerotic emboli, hypoperfusion, vasculitis), hereditary pancreatitis (mutations in trypsinogen gene) and idiopathic causes (10–25% of patients).

In this man alcohol can be excluded since he is a strict Muslim. Gallstone pancreatitis is the most likely diagnosis: this can occur at any age but is most common between the ages of 50 and 70 years. The diagnosis is often missed, ultrasound being only 70% to 80% sensitive in detecting gallstones during the acute phase of pancreatitis. Pancreatitis is a well recognised and important side effect of azathioprine.

Answer to Question 163
C

Non-alcoholic fatty liver disease (NAFLD) is a spectrum of diseases that includes simple steatosis, steatohepatitis, advanced fibrosis and cirrhosis. The diagnosis should be suspected in patients with persistently elevated alanine aminotransferase (ALT) values with negative screening for viral hepatitis, autoimmune hepatitis and metabolic liver disease, no high risk alcohol or medication use, and with fatty infiltration on ultrasound. NAFLD is associated with the metabolic syndrome (obesity, insulin resistance, hyperlipidaemia and hypertension) and is therefore often seen in obese patients who may have impaired glucose intolerance. Treatment and prognosis is unclear, but attention to modifiable risk factors is important, including weight loss, diabetic management and treatment of hyperlipidaemia.

Answer to Question 164
B

At first presentation or at the time of a subsequent flare of acute colitis it is always important to check stool cultures for standard bacterial pathogens including *Salmonella*, *Campylobacter* and *Shigella* as well as *Clostridium difficile*. However, in the context of severe disease it is not always possible to withhold steroids until negative cultures have been obtained, and steroid therapy does not appear to adversely affect outcome even when stool cultures come out positive. Indeed, infective colitis can trigger an episode of inflammatory bowel disease.

Clostridium difficile may produce characteristic pseudomembranes on macroscopic appearance but does not always do so. Differentiating CMV colitis from ulcerative colitis in which CMV inclusion bodies occur as "bystanders" is virtually impossible. Amoebic dysentery usually occurs in people living in or recently returned from the tropics but asymptomatic individuals can continue to excrete cysts for many years.

Answer to Question 165
B

Approximately 20% of patients with pseudomembranous colitis relapse, usually 2 weeks to 2 months after treatment. This is related to the persistence of *C.difficile* spores that are not killed by antibiotic therapy, rather than to metronidazole resistance, hence recurrence of disease should be treated with a second course of oral metronidazole. If he fails to respond to a second course of oral metronidazole then the second line agent would be oral (not intravenous) vancomycin.

Answer to Question 166
C

Campylobacter is the commonest cause of bacterial gastroenteritis in the UK, but its incubation period is three to five days. By contrast, the incubation period of *Salmonella* is eight to 48 hours. Treatment of *Salmonella* gastroenteritis is symptomatic. If the patient is very ill, then ciprofloxacin is the antibiotic of choice, but antibiotics prolong the duration of stool carriage and should not be given routinely.

Answer to Question 167
B

The most common symptoms of Crohn's disease are abdominal pain, often in the lower right quadrant, and diarrhoea. Rectal bleeding, weight loss and fever may also occur. Bleeding may be serious and persistent, leading to anaemia. Children with Crohn's disease may suffer delayed development and stunted growth. Long standing inflammation can result in stricture formation which may present as intermittent bowel obstruction. Markers of inflammation such as CRP or ESR are not necessarily significantly raised if the obstruction is due to fibrosis. Patients with small bowel strictures are advised to eat a low fibre diet to reduce the risk of food bolus obstruction.

Answer to Question 168
D

All patients who have diarrhoea and undergo flexible sigmoidoscopy or colonoscopy should have colon biopsies taken to exclude microscopic colitis, which is characterised by a normal appearance to the mucosa but a lymphocytic infiltration histologically. This condition is associated with NSAID use and unlike classical ulcerative colitis is rarely associated with toxic megacolon. Although cholestyramine and sulphasalazine have been used as treatment, budesonide is the only drug shown to be effective in a controlled clinical trial. Collagenous colitis overlaps with this condition in that the clinical symptoms are similar, but microscopically there is a layer of collagen beneath the submucosa rather than lymphocytic infiltration.

Answer to Question 169
C

Ulcerative colitis is most likely. An infectious colitis is less likely if the symptoms have been present for more than one week, but patients with acute severe colitis should be treated with oral ciprofloxacin to cover bacterial colitis until the diagnosis is clear. Ischaemic colitis would be very unusual at this age and as he was previously fit significant NSAID consumption is not likely.

Answer to Question 170
C

Nocturnal diarrhoea should not be attributed to IBS unless alternative causes have been very carefully and thoroughly investigated. The remaining features listed may be caused by other conditions but are all recognized as clinical presentations of Irritable Bowel Syndrome.

Answer to Question 171

D

These cases are difficult to manage. Ulcerative colitis is less likely to cause enterovesical fistulae than is Crohn's disease, so the fistula in this case is probably due to diverticular disease. Malignancy and ischaemia need also to be borne in mind. Treatment may be medical, surgical or a combination, but definitive surgery is usually favoured where possible. Diagnosis is best made in liaison with the urologists as well as gastrointestinal surgeons and often involves cystoscopy, CT scanning as well as careful lower GI investigations.

Answer to Question 172

B

Diverticula (usually acquired) are herniations of the mucosa and submucosa or the entire wall thickness through the muscle layer of any part of the gastrointestinal tract. The sigmoid colon is the most commonly affected segment (>95% of cases), although disease can involve the descending, ascending, and transverse colon as well as the jejunum, ileum, and duodenum. Acute diverticulitis results from the inspissation of faecal material in the neck of the diverticulum and resultant bacterial replication. Thereafter an abscess or peridiverticular inflammation occurs following rupture of a microscopic mucosal abscess into the mesentery. The infection may progress, fistulise, obstruct or spontaneously resolve.

Answer to Question 173

E

Malnutrition is common in hospital and impairs recovery from illness. This man is malnourished and recovering from major trauma: some form of nutritional support is necessary. His gastrointestinal tract seems to be working and hence short-term enteral nutrition is appropriate. Whilst supplements may be sufficient it is more likely that intensive nutrition via a naso-gastric tube is going to be needed to meet his increased nutritional demands. It is inappropriate to simply monitor him and, in view of a functioning gastrointestinal tract, not appropriate to choose parenteral nutrition. The nutrition is needed short-term and therefore a PEG tube is not required.

Answer to Question 174

C

A history of dysphagia to both liquids and solids is fairly typical for achalasia. The barium meal findings are consistent, though not diagnostic, and endoscopy has ruled out a peptic oesophageal stricture. Confirmation of the diagnosis is by oeosphageal manometry, which shows a high resting lower oesophageal sphincter pressure that fails to relax on swallowing. Anti-Ro/La antibodies are positive in scleroderma, which may affect the oesophagus causing dysmotility. Oesophageal candidiasis may occur in achalasia or diabetes, but the latter should not cause a dilated oesophagus. The Tensilon test is a diagnostic test for myasthenia gravis, which may present with difficulty swallowing.

Answer to Question 175

B

Reflux oesophagitis is very common and easily treated with simple postural measures and acid suppression. Most patients respond to treatment and there is no need to repeat endoscopy in every case. Severe disease, presence of oesophageal ulceration and follow up of Barrett's oesophagitis are reasonable indications for repeat endoscopy. There is no convincing evidence for routine Helicobacter eradication in this clinical situation and the lowest dose of acid suppression should be given when symptoms have settled, if any is required at all.

Answer to Question 176

A

This man has absolute dysphagia and needs to be in hospital. He may have a malignancy, a peptic stricture or a food bolus. Neurological or muscle disorders are less likely. Most would arrange early cautious upper GI endoscopy or failing that a gastrograffin swallow (risk of aspirating barium). If a malignant lesion is likely then further investigations are needed to determine the best treatment strategy. Options include stenting, chemoradiotherapy, PEG feeding (inserted either endoscopically or surgically) or palliation. Investigations such as CT, PET and endoscopic ultrasound allow staging of malignant disease and a multi-disciplinary approach to treatment is best.

Answer to Question 177

D

Pancreatic carcinoma classically causes painless jaundice, but the absence of pain does not exclude the diagnosis of gallstones. The other diagnoses listed can all cause jaundice but are much less likely to be the explanation in this case. If pancreatic cancer is the diagnosis, then liver blood tests are likely to reveal elevation of alkaline phosphatase (ALP) and gamma-glutamyl transpeptidase (GGT). Elevation of aspartate transaminase (AST) and alanine transaminase (ALT) will be less marked, and they may be normal. The key investigation is ultrasound, which is likely to reveal dilatation of intra- and extra-hepatic bile ducts. Endoscopic retrograde cholangiopancreatography (ERCP) or CT scanning should confirm the diagnosis.

Answer to Question 178
B

Poor dietary compliance accounts for most cases where there is a failure to improve on treatment. Ulcerative jejunitis, small bowel adenocarcinoma and an enteropathy-associated T cell lymphoma are recognised but rare complications and there is an association with pancreatic sufficiency.

Answer to Question 179
A

The presence of bacterial overgrowth in the small bowel is usually suspected on the result of a breath test. Bacterial fermentation of an oral dose of carbohydrate releases hydrogen, and of an oral dose of conjugated bile acid (with radiolabelled carbon in the amino portion) releases radiolabelled carbon dioxide. If there is an increase in bacteria in the upper small bowel, then an early peak in hydrogen or carbon dioxide can be detected in expired air. The diagnosis of bacterial overgrowth is confirmed if there are >100 000 mixed bacteria/ml in a duodenal aspirate. Small bowel enema will detect diverticula or strictures as a cause for overgrowth. Initial treatment is with 10 days of augmentin or tetracycline. Prolonged courses may be needed, and cyclical antibiotics for one week every four weeks may be used. Laparotomy/resection would only be contemplated if these manoeuvres failed, and if anatomical abnormality was confined to a relatively small segment of bowel.

Answer to Question 180
C

Giardia lamblia is a very common intestinal parasite and a frequent cause of diarrhoeal illness throughout the world. Although water remains the most common mode of transmission, there has been an increase in the number of person-to-person cases, especially related to children, as well as an increase in food-borne cases. Chronic diarrhoea and malabsorption are seen with persistent infection and since treatment is simple and effective, diagnosis

by duodenal biopsy is important. New antigen detection tests for stool may ultimately replace histology in some situations. The greatest clinical experience in treatment is with the nitroimidazole drugs, i.e. metronidazole, tinidazole, and ornidazole, which are highly effective. A 5- to 7-day course of metronidazole can be expected to cure over 90% of individuals, and a single dose of tinidazole or ornidazole will do likewise.

Answer to Question 181
E

When haemoglobin is broken down the porphyrin ring is converted into biliverdin and thence to bilirubin. Unconjugated bilirubin is relatively insoluble and is transported in the blood as a complex with albumin: it is not excreted in the urine. Hepatocytes take up unconjugated bilirubin and conjugate it to form the soluble diglucuronide, which is excreted into the bile. Further metabolism by gut bacteria forms the soluble colourless compound urobilinogen. Some of this enters the blood stream and is excreted in the urine. Urobilinogen remaining in the gut is converted to the brown pigment, urobilin, and is excreted. If a patient with jaundice has no urobilinogen in their urine, then they must have complete obstruction to bile flow.

Answer to Question 182
B

Bacterial fermentation of an oral dose of the carbohydrate lactulose releases hydrogen. If there is an increase in bacteria in the upper small bowel, or if there is rapid intestinal transit, then an early peak in hydrogen can be detected in expired air. An oral dose of conjugated bile acid, often glycine-glycocholate, with radiolabelled carbon in the amino portion, can be given as an alternative to lactulose. Bacterial action releases radiolabelled glycine, detected following metabolism as labelled carbon dioxide in the breath.

Neurology

Answer to Question 183
C

There is a left sixth nerve palsy: the left eye has adducted as appropriate for gaze to the left, but the right eye has not abducted at all, indeed it remains directed slightly to the right of the midline.

Answer to Question 184

D

There is gross cerebral atrophy, caused by Alzheimer's disease in this case. The lateral ventricles are markedly dilated, but this appearance is caused by 'shrinkage' of the brain. Look at the cortical sulci: these are very large; in hydrocephalus they would be almost obliterated.

Answer to Question 185

C, J

Cerebellar lesion can be acute or chronic, symmetrical or asymmetric, isolated or part of a more widespread degenerative condition. The symptoms are characteristically worse in the dark and can come on slowly in degenerative conditions. Headache and double vision are common in pontine-cerebellar lesion. On examination the classical findings are horizontal nystagmus, with gait and limb ataxia. The finding of papilloedema suggests a posterior fossa space-occupying lesion and upgoing plantars may be indicative of a brain stem lesion. Very brief symptoms associated with head movement are more suggestive of benign paroxysmal positional vertigo (BPPV); neck pain and wasting of hand muscles raise the possibility of a cervical myelopathy.

Answer to Question 186

D, H

A transient ischaemic attack (TIA) is defined as an episode of acute loss of focal cerebral or monocular function lasting less than 24 hours. Since any signs will almost certainly have disappeared before the patient is assessed, the diagnosis depends entirely upon the history. Non-focal symptoms such as loss of consciousness, dizziness, mental confusion, generalised weakness and incontinence are not acceptable as evidence of TIA. In addition, some focal signs occurring in isolation should not be interpreted as TIA because they can so often mislead. These include vertigo, diplopia, dysphagia, dysphonia, loss of balance, tinnitus, amnesia and sensory symptoms with restricted distribution.

Answer to Question 187

G, J

Non-epileptic attacks can usually be distinguished fairly reliably on clinical grounds, but difficulty often arises with frontal lobe seizures that can be bizarre and occur without EEG change. Cyanosis and repetitive chewing movements are suggestive of epileptic seizures. Recovery usually occurs over a few minutes rather than immediately. Carpet burns, opisthotonus and pelvic thrusting are classically associated with non-epileptic attacks. Tongue-biting is seen with both types of attack and is non-discriminatory.

Answer to Question 188

C, F

Guillain–Barré classically presents with an ascending paralysis beginning in the legs. Sensory involvement is variable, but usually less than motor features. Reflexes are lost early in the illness. Demyelinating neuropathies characteristically cause fatigue with repeated use. The cranial nerves are commonly affected, most commonly the facial nerves. The autonomic nerves can be involved leading to pupillary abnormalities and haemodynamic instability. The bladder and bowel can be affected, but early involvement would be more suggestive of a conus lesion. Guillain–Barré is very painful, and can present with back pain.

Answer to Question 189

C

The diagnosis in this case is juvenile myoclonic epilepsy (JME) and sodium valproate is the treatment of choice. The chance of seizure recurrence with this type of epilepsy is high so treatment is warranted. Phenytoin and carbamazepine are useful only for partial seizures or generalised tonic-clonic seizures: they are ineffective (and may worsen) myoclonic jerks and absence seizures. Gabapentin is licensed only for use in partial epilepsy. Clonazepam is effective treatment for myoclonic jerks but less effective and more sedating than sodium valproate in absences and generalised tonic-clonic seizures. An alternative to valproate in JME, particularly in women of child-bearing age, is lamotrigine.

Answer to Question 190

E

Benign essential tremor is a fine tremor that often starts in childhood or adolescence but only presents later when it becomes functionally debilitating. The tremor is typically worse on using the affected limb, e.g. using a knife and fork or holding a cup. It can be sporadic or inherited as an autosomal dominant with variable penetrance. The tremor is improved by alcohol. Tremor is rarely the only symptom of cerebellar disease and gait disorder would certainly be present if tremor was caused by cerebellar disorder.

Answer to Question 191

C

Parkinson's disease is typically asymmetrical at presentation. The tremor is worst at rest, hence it is usually possible for the patient to drink, unlike benign essential tremor where action makes the tremor worse. Marked chewing movements and lip-smacking suggest drug-induced Parkinsonism and an extended neck and raised eyebrows suggest progressive supranuclear palsy; the neck is characteristically flexed in Parkinson's disease. A positive glabellar tap is common in normal older people and is not useful as a diagnostic sign.

Answer to Question 192

D

New variant Creutzfeldt-Jakob disease (CJD) commonly presents in young adults with psychiatric symptoms followed by non-specific painful sensory symptoms, most often in the lower limbs. Cognitive impairment, pyramidal signs, myoclonus and primitive reflexes then develop. Mean disease duration is approximately 14 months. MRI commonly shows high signal on T2-weighted images in the pulvinar (posterior aspect of thalamus). EEG is often normal, compared to sporadic CJD in which triphasic waves are observed. Diagnosis is made ante-mortem by brain biopsy or more commonly tonsillar biopsy. The CSF contains 14-3-3 protein which is clearly linked with bovine spongiform encephalopathy (BSE).

Answer to Question 193

D

A high stepping gait is most likely to be due to bilateral foot drop.

Answer to Question 194

D

Multiple sclerosis typically presents at an earlier age (<50 years) and produces upper motor neurone signs only, i.e. no wasting or fasciculation. Miller–Fisher is a variant of Guillain–Barré syndrome and presents with ataxia, areflexia and ophthalmoplegia. Basilar artery thrombosis is an acute event, often with obtundation, mixed cranial nerve dysfunction and long tract signs. Wernicke's encephalopathy presents with gaze palsies, and cognitive impairment. Amyotrophic lateral sclerosis is characterised by a combination of upper and lower motor neurone abnormalities: 20% of patients present with bulbar onset.

Answer to Question 195

E

She is likely to have spinal cord compression from metastases. Plain radiographs and CT may give some information but the imaging modality of choice is MRI. Lumbar puncture and myelography carry the risk of clinical deterioration.

Answer to Question 196

C

L4 is involved in knee extension and ankle inversion.

Answer to Question 197

C

C5/C6 supplies the following muscles: deltoid, biceps, brachioradialis, supra and infra spinati, pectoralis major (clavicular head), serratus anterior (causes winging of scapula if weak), extensor carpi radialis longus. Both biceps and brachioradialis reflexes may be affected in a C5/C6 lesion. Sensory loss can be variable but typically involves the lateral (radial) aspect of the upper and lower arm including the thumb. C8 typically supplies the ring and little finger.

Answer to Question 198

E

The patient has cluster headache. Prophylactic treatments that can be used include verapamil, prednisolone, lithium carbonate, ergotamine and methysergide.

Answer to Question 199

A

The signs described here are cortical sensory signs and indicative of a lesion of the anterior parietal cortex, particularly mid postcentral gyrus.

Answer to Question 200

D

Guillain-Barré syndrome is preceded by respiratory or gastrointestinal symptoms in two-thirds, but not all, cases. Lower back pain, often radiating to the buttocks, occurs in 20–30% of cases and results in an incorrect diagnosis of lumbar vertebral or disc disease being made in many cases. Difficulty walking in this case is due to distal weakness as suggested by the history of difficulty walking or tripping on uneven ground. This, together with the probable areflexia, suggest a peripheral neuropathy of acute onset. Acute transverse myelitis may be very difficult to distinguish in the first few days before upper motor neuron signs develop.

Answer to Question 201

C

L2, 3 radiates to the anterior thigh. L5 radiates through the buttock, down the posteriolateral aspect of the thigh, lateral aspect of calf and across the dorsum of the foot to the big toe. S1 radiates through the inner buttock to the posterior aspect of the thigh, posteriolateral aspect of the calf to the lateral border of the foot.

Answer to Question 202

B

A relative afferent pupillary defect (RAPD) is detected using the 'swinging light test'. It allows comparison of pupillary constriction generated through the afferent pathway (within the retina or optic nerve anterior to the chiasm) of each eye with that produced consensually. After checking for direct and consensual pupillary responses in each eye, proceed as follows. Shine a bright light into the right eye for five seconds. Look at the pupil of the left eye. Move the light swiftly to shine in the left eye. If the left pupil dilates, there is a left RAPD. Now observe the pupil of the right eye. Move the light back to the right eye. If the right pupil dilates there is a right RAPD.

Answer to Question 203

D

A common peroneal nerve lesion leads to foot drop with loss of ankle and toe dorsiflexion and ankle eversion. Numbness occurs over the lateral aspect of the lower leg and dorsum of the foot. It is usually due to pressure over the fibular head. An L5 root lesion causes weakness of ankle dorsiflexion, inversion and eversion and dorsiflexion of the great toe. Numbness occurs down the posteriolateral aspect of the thigh, lateral aspect of the calf and across the dorsum of the foot to the great toe. Loss of the ankle jerk occurs in lesions of S1.

Ophthalmology

Answer to Question 204

B

The appearance of the disc is consistent with either optic neuritis or papilloedema, but in the latter visual acuity would not be impaired.

Answer to Question 205

C

The fundus shows the characteristic 'bloodstorm' appearance and cotton-wool spots of central retinal vein occlusion.

Answer to Question 206

A

Visual impairment more marked for reading than distance is very suggestive of macular disease, and the likely cause of symptoms in this case is diabetic maculopathy, when the central fovea becomes affected by retinal oedema or frank hard exudate. Age-related macular degeneration would be unlikely in a man of this age.

Answer to Question 207

C

All of the preparations listed can be used to dilate the pupils, but tropicamide (0.5% for children, 1% for adults) is best for diagnostic purposes, dilating the pupil for two to four hours by blocking the parasympathetic terminals in the papillary constrictor muscle. Cyclopentolate works in a similar manner but lasts for six to eight hours.

Phenylephrine drops dilate the pupil by stimulating the sympathetic system. They should be used with caution both in children and in adults with ischaemic heart disease because they can induce hypertension, exacerbate angina or induce arrhythmias.

Psychiatry

Answer to Question 208

D, I

The most common aetiological factors in HIV/AIDS-associated psychotic disorders are prexisiting psychotic disorders, substance misuse, psychogenic reaction, iatrogenic factors and HIV related brain disease.

Answer to Question 209

D

A wide range of biochemical/haematological abnormalities can be found in anorexia nervosa. These include hypokalaemia, hypochloraemic alkalosis (both due to vomiting and/or diuretic/laxative abuse) and hypercholesterolaemia (mechanism unknown). The ESR is normal or reduced.

Answer to Question 210

B

Lewy body dementia is characterised by fluctuating cognition, visual hallucinations, parkinsonism, neuroleptic sensitivity, falls/transient loss of consciousness/syncope and delusions. Vascular dementia typically occurs in those with widespread vascular disease. The course is typically fluctuating with stepwise progression. Differentiation from Alzheimer's disease can be difficult.

Answer to Question 211

E

Chronic fatigue syndrome is defined as clinically evaluated, medically unexplained fatigue of at least six months' duration that is of new onset, not a result of ongoing exertion, not substantially alleviated by rest, and leads to a substantial reduction in previous levels of activity. Four or more of the following symptoms are also required for diagnosis: subjective memory impairment, tender lymph nodes, muscle pain, joint pain, headache, unrefreshing sleep and postexertional malaise.

Endocrinology

Answer to Question 212

B

The left eye has failed to abduct due to a left sixth nerve palsy. The sclerae can be seen above the iris of both eyes indicating the presence of lid retraction. Lid lag is demonstrated by asking the patient to look at an object moved from superior to inferior in the visual field and cannot be determined from a still photograph of a patient attempting to look to the left.

Answer to Question 213

A

The absence of facial hair and the fine wrinkles around the corners of the eyes and mouth make hypogonadism the most likely diagnosis. A low serum testosterone level will confirm the diagnosis, and measurement of LH and FSH allows distinction between hypogonadotrophic and hypergonadotrophic causes. Hypogonadotrophic causes, where the testicular problem is secondary to pituitary/hypothalamic dysfunction, include constitutional delayed puberty, hyperprolactinaemia, pituitary tumour / infiltra-tion / radiation / surgery, Kallman's syndrome and idiopathic. Hypergonadotrophic causes, where the testicular problem is primary, include post chemotherapy / viral / trauma, Klinefelter's syndrome, systemic disorders (e.g. renal failure) and idiopathic.

Answer to Question 214

A

The radiograph (Figure 30) shows Looser's zones caused by pseudofractures in a patient with severe osteomalacia. Although a definitive diagnosis of this condition can only be made by bone biopsy, this is rarely justified, the combination of low / low-normal serum calcium, low / low-normal serum phosphate and elevated serum alkaline phosphate being sufficient in an appropriate clinical context. Note that levels of 1,25-dihydroxy-vitamin D are often within the 'normal range', but this is inappropriate in the face of hypocalcaemia, hypophosphataemia and secondary hyperparathyroidism.

Answer to Question 215

B, G

Primary and tertiary hyperparathyroidism will cause hypercalcaemia, whereas secondary hyperparathyroidism is caused by overactivity of the parathyroid glands to compensate for long standing hypocalcaemia and does not result in elevated calcium levels. Any granulomatous disease can cause hypercalcaemia, including sarcoidosis, berylliosis and tuberculosis.

Answer to Question 216

G, J

This woman has osteomalacia with secondary hyperparathyroidism developing because of chronic vitamin D deficiency and associated hypocalcaemia. Patients with primary hyperparathyroidism, ectopic PTH production (e.g. from lung cancer) or bony metastases will usually have hypercalcaemia. Her renal function is grossly normal and the low calcium and fairly low phosphate rule out tertiary hyperparathyroidism. Patients with uncomplicated Paget's disease and osteoporosis usually have normal calcium and PTH levels. A high level of PTH excludes post-thyroidectomy hypocalcaemia. In pseudohypoparathyroidism, PTH resistance leads to high circulating PTH, with high phosphate and low calcium, sometimes in association with multiple bony abnormalities. In pseudopseudohypoparathyroidism these bony abnormalities occur without any derangement of calcium levels.

Answer to Question 217
B, E

The key components of the MEN1 syndrome are parathyroid hyperplasia, pancreatic tumours (e.g. gastrinoma, insulinoma) and pituitary tumours (most commonly prolactinomas). Although carcinoid tumours occur in a small number (3–5%) of patients with MEN1, routine screening with urinary 5-HIAA is not generally advocated in asymptomatic individuals. Measurement of a random plasma glucose level is not a useful means of screening for the presence of an insulinoma, a diagnosis that should be based on Whipple's triad of biochemical hypoglycaemia with symptoms that are relieved by administration of glucose. Despite the history of prior 'total' parathyroidectomy it is necessary to periodically monitor serum calcium levels to ensure adequacy of replacement with vitamin D/calcium supplements, and in case the individual harbours an additional ectopically sited gland that could result in a relapse.

Medullary thyroid carcinoma (calcitonin) and phaeochromocytoma (urinary catecholamines) are typically associated with the MEN2 syndrome.

Answer to Question 218
G, H

Amiodarone-induced thyroid dysfunction is a common problem in endocrine practice. As amiodarone interferes with deiodinase, free T4, free T3 and TSH should be considered together (high fT4 may be associated with low cellular fT3 levels). Amiodarone contains in excess of 35% iodine by weight and in patients with autoimmune subclinical hypothyroidism this may be sufficient to suppress thyroid function (the Wolff-Chaikov effect) leading to clinical hypothyroidism in about 6% of patients in iodine-replete populations. By contrast, in iodine deficiency Graves' hyperthyroidism may be unmasked by sudden amiodarone (iodine) loading (type 1 amiodarone-induced thyrotoxicosis, the Jod-Basedow effect) and autonomy can develop in nodular goiters to drive thyrotoxicosis once iodine is replaced. Type 2 amiodarone-induced thyrotoxicosis is the result of inflammatory destruction of thyroid tissue and release of preformed hormone. This condition requires the initial use of high dose steroids to suppress it, and is most commonly associated with reduced or absent signal on scintigraphy. Thyroid ultrasonography with colour flow Doppler may be useful in distinguishing the absent vascular signal of type 2 from the normal or increased vascularity of type 1 thyrotoxicosis.

Answer to Question 219
E

$2 \times (Na + K) + urea + glucose$ = approximation of serum osmolality, with the normal range being 285 to 295 mOsm/l. In hyperglycaemic hyperosmolar non-ketotic syndrome plasma osmolality is >320 mOsm/Kg and blood glucose >33 mmol/l.

Answer to Question 220
B

This woman has hypoparathyroidism. Patients with pseudohypoparathyroidism have somatic features and PTH levels are high because of target organ resistance. Patients with pseudopseudohypoparathyroidism have the somatic features without biochemical abnormality. Renal failure is excluded by normal urea and creatinine.

It is difficult to differentiate between idiopathic hypoparathyroidism and the familial / autoimmune hypoparathyroidism that occurs as a part of polyglandular autoimmune syndrome type 1. However, without any family history of autoimmune disorder and without any personal history of problems such as mucocutaneous candidiasis, vitiligo or alopecia, this woman's hypocalcaemia is most likely to be due to idiopathic / acquired hypoparathyroidism.

Answer to Question 221
C

This patient's clinical picture is very suggestive of a pituitary adenoma, although it is difficult on the information given to ascertain whether he has a secretory or a non-secretory tumour. High prolactin levels may be seen in prolactinomas or any other pituitary or non-pituitary tumours where pressure from the tumour mass on the pituitary stalk functionally disconnects the inhibitory input from the hypothalamus. Some growth hormone secreting adenomas also secrete prolactin. Low levels of some pituitary hormones occur due to local effects of the pituitary adenoma (whether secretory or non-secretory). Secondary hypothyroidism due to lack of thyroid-stimulating hormone (TSH), adrenocortical deficiency due to lack of adrenocorticotropic hormone (ACTH), low IGF-1 associated with growth hormone deficiency, and low testosterone associated with FSH and LH deficiency (hypogonadotrophic hypogonadism) can all occur together, in different combinations, or on their own.

Answer to Question 222

D

Plasma ADH concentration is normally controlled by plasma osmolality, but pain, nausea, hypovolaemia and anaesthesia are all powerful stimulants of ADH release and can generate much higher plasma levels than are seen in response to tonicity. Nausea and hypovolaemia are likely to have stimulated very high ADH levels as the explanation for this man's hyponatraemia. In recognition of these facts, SIADH can only be diagnosed when the following criteria are satisfied: the patient is clinically euvolaemic (JVP seen, no postural hypotension); decreased plasma sodium concentration and osmolality; inappropriately high urinary sodium concentration (>20 mmol/l) and osmolality (>plasma); there is normal adrenal, thyroid and renal function.

Answer to Question 223

A

Growth hormone (GH) secretion is pulsatile, hence a single random GH level is not a reliable assessment of GH secretion. After 75 g of oral glucose suppression of GH to <1 mU/l excludes the diagnosis of acromegaly. Once the diagnosis is established, imaging of the pituitary fossa (preferably by MRI) can distinguish micro- from macro-adenomas. Visual acuity, visual fields and anterior pituitary function also require formal assessment.

Answer to Question 224

C

Whilst GH has some direct actions (e.g. antagonism of insulin), many of its effects are mediated through IGF-1, which is produced by the liver and, accordingly, in acro-megaly IGF-1 levels are typically elevated above the age- and sex-related reference range.

Unless the GH level is dramatically elevated, the diagnosis of acromegaly should not be made on the basis of a single random GH measurement – if sampling coincides with a normal physiological 'spike' in GH secretion a false positive result may ensue.

Most cases of acromegaly (approximately 75%) arise in the setting of a pituitary macroadenoma (>1 cm in diameter). These tumours may encroach on the optic chiasm, classically resulting in a bitemporal visual field defect. In addition, the remaining normal anterior pituitary tissue is often compressed – in these circumstances one might expect the gonadotrophin levels to fall within or below the reference range for younger females, which would of course be inappropriate in the post-menopausal state, where the gonadotrophins are typically elevated.

Answer to Question 225

B

The first line treatment is usually surgery, with trans-sphenoidal adenectomy curing 80% of patients with microadenomas and 50% of those with macroadenomas. Somatostatin analogues are effective symptomatically in 60% of cases and produce a significant reduction in tumour size in 30%, but they can only be given as injections, are expensive, and have a number of side effects. Dopamine antagonists are of very limited efficacy, although they can be useful if the tumour co-secretes prolactin.

Answer to Question 226

B

It appears that she either has a prolactinoma or there is some other pituitary tumour affecting her pituitary stalk. There is also evidence of hypopituitarism as reflected by lack of TSH response to a low level of thyroxine. It is quite possible that she may have adrenocortical deficiency secondary to lack of adrenocorticotropic hormone (ACTH) as well as other pituitary deficiencies and mandatory to either exclude adrenocortical insufficiency or, in emergency situations, to give glucocorticoids before starting thyroxine. Replacing thyroxine in the face of untreated adrenocortical deficiency can lead to life-threatening adrenal crisis. She will need an MRI scan of the pituitary gland and also some other pituitary hormone assays / provocative tests, but the most important test at this point is a short tetracosactide (Synacthen) test for a quick assessment of hypothalamo-pituitary-adrenal axis. Ultimately treatment may be with cabergoline (or similar) if prolactinoma is confirmed.

Answer to Question 227

C

Growth hormone (GH) deficiency is associated with loss of lean body mass, increase in fat mass, hyperlipidaemia, increased risk of osteoporosis, and cardiovascular morbidity and mortality. Treatment with GH in adults is controversial and many clinicians only consider it in patients who are symptomatic in addition to being biochemically GH deficient. This is because GH is relatively expensive and as yet there is no hard end-point data on reduction of cardiovascular adverse events or osteoporotic fractures. Several studies have shown improvement in surrogate markers of these diseases, including markers of bone turnover and plasma lipids. Wellbeing scores and exercise tolerance have also been shown to improve, hence the concentration on symptomatic patients. Although there is a theoretical concern about promoting tumour growth, the dose of GH is titrated against IGF-1 to prevent over-replacement. So far there is no evidence to suggest an increased risk of new tumour formation or recurrence of a previously treated pituitary tumour.

Answer to Question 228
D

This woman is hypothyroid and has presumably experienced an early menopause, together suggestive either of pituitary disease or autoimmune polyglandular disease. The presentation with headache, third and sixth nerve palsies, and refractory hypotension suggests pituitary disease, such as a macroprolactinoma, complicated by infarction or haemorrhage. In this situation the key is to consider the diagnosis and administer adequate intravenous steroid (e.g. 100 mg hydrocortisone) to facilitate resuscitation before emergency MRI imaging to look for pituitary haemorrhage and mass effect. Emergency transphenoidal debulking may be necessary. Failure to demonstrate pituitary pathology should lead to angiography to look for a berry aneurysm.

Answer to Question 229
B

According to guidelines from the Royal College of Physicians, men and women over the age of 65 who are on chronic (more than 3 months) steroid therapy should be started on treatment such as antiresorptive drugs to prevent osteoporosis. They should go onto such therapy at the same time as they commence steroids. A DEXA scan is not required as they need preventive therapy regardless of the result such a scan might show. HRT may have a limited role early in the postmenopausal period, but only for a limited time and mainly for vasomotor symptoms. At the age of 66 HRT is not recommended for osteoporosis prevention therapy.

Answer to Question 230
C

The pathogenesis of corticosteroid induced osteoporosis is multifactorial. Corticosteroids reduce osteoblastic activity and the resulting osteoblast / osteoclast imbalance causes loss of bone. They also reduce intestinal calcium absorption and lower circulating sex steroid levels. Corticosteroid induced bone loss is fastest in the first 3–6 months of therapy.

Answer to Question 231
C

The treatment of choice for Paget's disease is intravenous infusion of sodium pamidronate. A single dose of 60 mg can produce remission for six months or longer in mild or limited Paget's disease: those with more extensive disease require multiple doses. Alendronate is approved in the United States and risendronate and tiludronate are undergoing trials.

There is an increased risk of osteosarcoma and pathological fracture in Paget's disease, hence radiological investigation is needed to exclude these pathologies in a patient with increased bone pain.

Answer to Question 232
C

Hypercalcaemia and primary hyperparathyroidism are recognised side effects of long-term treatment with lithium in subjects with chronic affective psychiatric disorders. It has been suggested that lithium alters the sensitivity of the parathyroid cells to calcium and leads to hyperplasia. However, other studies have failed to confirm an excess of parathyroid hyperplasia in this population, suggesting instead that lithium selectively stimulates the growth of parathyroid adenomas in susceptible patients, who are best treated with excision of the adenoma rather than total parathyroidectomy.

Answer to Question 233
C

The patient has significant renal impairment, PTH is raised, calcium is raised and so is phosphate: the diagnosis is tertiary hyperparathyroidism. Primary hyperparathyroidism causes low phosphate levels and rarely leads to PTH levels as high as in this case. The raised calcium excludes secondary hyperparathyroidism, since calcium is normal and PTH raised in this condition. Exogenous replacement therapy (unless delivered in primary hyperparathyroidism) should suppress PTH.

Answer to Question 234
D

Constitutional delay is common in boys and by far the commonest cause of short stature with delayed pubertal development. Diagnosis requires there to be no pubertal development by the age of 14 in boys (13 in girls, in whom the condition is much less common) and for the bone age to be at least 3 years less than the chronological age (showing that there is still potential for growth). The condition may not require treatment other than reassurance that puberty and increased growth will eventually occur, along with follow-up to monitor growth. However, if the condition is causing distress, puberty can be accelerated by treatment with testosterone to prime the hypothalamo-pituitary-gonadal axis.

Coeliac disease and other chronic illnesses can also cause delayed puberty, but this would be a less common cause and you might expect there to be other associated symptoms or signs. Growth hormone deficiency in childhood is much rarer than constitutional delayed puberty and presents with failure of linear growth at any age, rather than the characteristic normal growth followed by falling behind as peers undergo their pubertal growth spurt described above. Kleinfelter's syndrome (47XXY) is associated with primary hypogonadism (i.e. testicular failure) whilst Kallman's syndrome is characterised by secondary (hypogonadotrophic) hypogonadism with anosmia. Both conditions are generally associated with tall rather than short stature.

Answer to Question 235

E

If endogenous insulin were the cause, whether generated by a tumour (insulinoma) or in response to stimulation by an oral hypoglycaemic agent, then levels of insulin and C-peptide would both be elevated. The only thing that can produce dissociation between insulin and C-peptide levels is administration of exogenous insulin.

Answer to Question 236

D

Long-term carbimazole is an option, but dose requirement is high and she may run into side effects. Giving another dose of radioactive iodine is simpler, quite likely to be successful and may be curative. Surgery is also an option, but in a frail patient it would be standard practice to try at least one further dose of radioactive iodine before considering this. Propylthiouracil has no advantage over carbimazole. Block and replace therapy is not used in this clinical situation.

Nephrology

Answer to Question 237

D

The appearances of the arm are consistent with crush injury. If perfusion or sensation in the hand is impaired then urgent orthopaedic opinion is required: fasciotomy or debridement may save the limb. The expected cause of renal failure in this scenario is rhabdomyolysis, which leads to urine that tests strongly positive for blood on stick testing but contains no red cells on microscopy (because the stick test is detecting the presence of myoglobin from crushed muscle), gross elevation of the serum creatine kinase, and is often associated with hyperkalaemia.

Answer to Question 238

E

This man is clearly extremely unwell. The differential diagnosis is wide, but the two most likely diagnoses are bacterial pneumonia and relapse of Wegener's. It will certainly be appropriate to urgently check the titre of anti-neutrophil cytoplasmic antibodies (ANCA), also to send blood and sputum cultures, and investigation of the chest with CT scan, respiratory function tests (looking for raised kCO suggestive of pulmonary haemorrhage) and bronchoscopy may be needed. However, in this scenario it may well be fatal to delay treatment of treatable causes, so 'shoot first and ask questions afterwards' is the correct course of action in this case.

Answer to Question 239

C

Figure 33 shows three glomeruli, two of which are clearly abnormal, hence the disease is focal, meaning that it affects some glomeruli and not others. The glomeruli that are affected contain some areas (segments) that are abnormal and some areas that are not, hence the condition is segmental. Within the parts of the glomeruli that are diseased there are amorphous areas that appear pink with this Haematoxylin and Eosin stain, which is characteristic of necrotic tissue. In summary, the biopsy shows focal, segmental, necrotizing glomerulonephritis, which is characteristic of microscopic polyangiitis.

Answer to Question 240

C, G

Thiazide diuretics and loop diuretics such as bumetanide promote renal potassium loss and can cause hypokalaemia.

Aldosterone enhances sodium reabsorption and potassium secretion in the distal nephron, hence conditions such as Conn's syndrome or Cushing's disease or steroid therapy in which there is excess mineralocorticoid activity are associated with hypokalaemia. In Addison's disease there is a deficiency of aldosterone and a tendency to hyperkalaemia. Spironolactone has a similar effect because it antagonises the action of aldosterone. Activation of the renin angiotensin axis promotes aldosterone production, which can happen in renal artery stenosis or accelerated phase hypertension.

Answer to Question 241

B, C

The patient has bilateral upper tract obstruction for which the most likely causes are retroperitoneal fibrosis, lymphoma or malignant infiltration. A CT scan will define the site of the obstruction and narrow the list of probable causes. Nephrostomies will be appropriate in the short term. If the diagnosis is retroperitoneal fibrosis, moderate dose oral steroids will be indicated for the systemic symptoms. Although surgical ureterolysis may be performed, ureteric stents are often a very satisfactory treatment. Once obstruction is relieved the patient is likely to be polyuric, and the prognosis for recovery of renal function is good given preserved cortical thickness. Bladder catheterisation is not indicated.

Answer to Question 242

C, G

The major abnormalities are hypocalcaemia and hyperphosphataemia secondary to chronic renal failure. In chronic renal failure there is failure of the renal 1-alpha hydroxylase enzyme, preventing vitamin D from being converted to 1-alpha hydroxycholecalciferol, an intermediary on the way to the main active metabolite, 1,25-dihydroxycholecalciferol. Hypercalcaemia can therefore be corrected with 1-alpha hydroxycholecalciferol, which should be done to prevent/retard the development of secondary hyperparathyroidism that has long-term adverse consequences, particularly on bone. In chronic renal failure there is also phosphate retention that can be ameliorated by the consumption of phosphate binders before/at the same time as food. Calcium carbonate is commonly used. Aluminium hydroxide is also effective, but is no longer used (except in rare circumstances) because of the adverse consequences of aluminium intoxication. Sevelamer is an effective alternative.

Answer to Question 243

B

Aldosterone enhances distal nephron sodium reabsorption, causing fluid retention and/or hypertension depending on the clinical context, and increased potassium secretion in the collecting tubules, leading to potassium depletion. Hypertension can cause glomerular damage, hence a trace of proteinuria is a common finding in hypertensive patients. Minimal change nephropathy presents with nephrotic syndrome. Mesangiocapillary glomerulonephritis can cause hypertension but would be associated with much heavier proteinuria than that described.

Answer to Question 244

D

There is clear evidence that angiotensin converting enzyme inhibition in diabetics delays progression of renal failure, even if they are normotensive by conventional criteria. A loop diuretic will improve the peripheral oedema but there is no evidence that it would preserve renal function. Cholesterol lowering is appropriate given the patient's vascular risk factors but it does not alter the progression of renal disease.

Answer to Question 245

A

It is typically 10–20 years after the diagnosis of type I diabetes mellitus that patients first experience microalbuminuria, then heavier proteinuria, followed by renal functional decline. The development of renal failure has occurred too soon in this case to be ascribed to diabetic renal disease, and the fact that significant proteinuria did not precede renal impairment is also atypical. About one third of patients with diabetic nephropathy progress through a nephrotic phase, but this patient will require a renal biopsy to establish a precise diagnosis.

Answer to Question 246

B

This is a classic presentation of non-diarrhoeal haemolytic uraemic syndrome (D-HUS) or atypical HUS. This may be sporadic or familial. In sporadic cases association with HIV, malignancy, systemic lupus erythematosus (SLE) and some drugs (e.g. ciclosporin) has been reported. In some familial cases mutations have been detected in Factor H, which regulates the alternative pathway activation of complement. Thrombotic thrombocytopenic purpura (TTP) can produce a similar picture, but neurological involvement predominates. There is also evidence that the mechanism underlying the disease is different, with reduced activity of a von Willebrand factor cleaving protease ADAMTS13 in TTP but not in HUS. Treatment of sporadic HUS is with plasma exchange and fresh frozen plasma. The renal outlook is poor and mortality around 10%.

Answer to Question 247
C

Angiotensin II has a number of actions on the kidney. It is a vasoconstrictor, but its effect on the efferent arterioles is greater than that on the afferent arterioles, resulting in an increase in glomerular filtration rate. It also promotes sodium reabsorption in the proximal tubule by an action on sodium/hydrogen exchange at this site. Angiotensin II stimulates aldosterone release from the adrenal gland. Aldosterone promotes distal tubular sodium reabsorption and potassium secretion. Angiotensin-converting enzyme (ACE) inhibitors block the effects of angiotensin II by inhibiting its formation, hence glomerular filtration rate often falls slightly and aldosterone levels fall. The fall in aldosterone reduces sodium reabsorption in the distal tubule and the fall in angiotensin II reduces sodium reabsorption in the proximal tubule. Conversely, the fall in aldosterone reduces distal tubular potassium secretion and so serum potassium concentration can rise.

Answer to Question 248
D

Rhabdomyolysis results from muscle injury and the release of myoglobin from muscle cells. Myoglobin is toxic to the renal tubules and oliguria or even anuria can occur. Myoglobinuria usually occurs. Muscle cells also release creatine kinase and potassium when they are injured. Red cell casts are not a feature of rhabdomyolysis and would suggest glomerulonephritis or vasculitis as the cause of his acute renal failure.

Answer to Question 249
B

Hydroxylated vitamin D suppresses PTH expression and alfacalcidol should be considered for prophylaxis against renal bone disease and progressive hyperparathyroidism. However, the obvious abnormality is that the patient's serum phosphate level is elevated and the priority must be to reduce this. Calcium acetate would be the most reasonable choice of phosphate binder here: it should be

taken with (or just before) meals and may offer advantages over calcium carbonate, especially in patients with reduced gastric acidity. Aluminium-containing phosphate binders carry the risk of aluminium accumulation and neurological side effects and are no longer used (except in rare instances). Sevelamer is only clearly indicated if calcium-containing binders cannot be used because the calcium level (or calcium-phosphate product) are undesirably high. Parathyroidectomy is not indicated: the patient only has a mildly elevated level of PTH that is likely to improve with better phosphate control.

Answer to Question 250
C

The patient has nephrotic syndrome and at this age the commonest underlying diagnosis is minimal change nephrotic syndrome. This would also be consistent with the sudden onset, lack of haematuria and normal excretory renal function.

Thin membrane nephropathy presents with asymptomatic haematuria. IgA nephropathy can present with nephrotic syndrome, but this would be most unusual. Mesangiocapillary glomerulonephrits or membranous nephropathy can present with nephrotic syndrome but are much less common than minimal change disease at this age.

Answer to Question 251
D

Urinary stones made of calcium oxalate or of cystine are radio-opaque and would be visible on a plain radiograph: by contrast, those made of uric acid are radiolucent. Adult polycystic kidney disease does not cause renal colic, excepting very rarely if severe haematuria leads to clot colic, and the ultrasound finding would be of cysts, which do not cast acoustic shadows. Patients with uric acid stones always excrete acid urine. Once the acute problem is dealt with, if necessary by urological intervention, it will be important to advise this man to drink enough to ensure a urinary volume of at least 2 litres/day and to prescribe sufficient alkali (sodium or potassium bicarbonate) to achieve urinary pH > 6.2.

Answer to Question 252
E

The practice of double micturition endeavours to make sure that the bladder is completely empty after voiding, making it more difficult for infection to take hold. The woman should be advised to empty her bladder, wait for a further 60 seconds on the toilet and then try to void again. Some find that pressing on the suprapubic region helps to express more urine. Cranberry juice has antiseptic properties and has been shown in a controlled trial to be effective at reducing risk of urinary tract infection.

Answer to Question 253

A

The calcium x phosphate product is high, putting the patient at risk of metastatic calcification. Lowering the phosphate (rather than the calcium) is the most important measure as the elevated phosphate stimulates parathyroid proliferation and PTH secretion. This is best done by reinforcing dietary restriction and ensuring that the patient is receiving adequate dialysis. The vitamin D analogue will be increasing absorption of calcium and phosphate, so this should be reduced or stopped; ideally the patient will remain on a small dose as this helps to stop parathyroid proliferation. If these changes do not return the calcium and phosphate to satisfactory values, the patient should be changed to a phosphate binder that does not contain calcium. Aluminium based compounds are best avoided because of the risk of toxicity, hence sevelamer would be an appropriate (but expensive) choice.

Answer to Question 254

D

Probenecid is a uricosuric agent and will produce very little (if any) benefit in a patient with severe renal impairment necessitating haemodialysis. Allopurinol, if tolerated, will reduce urate production, and increased dialysis will improve urate clearance, both reducing the serum urate level and thus the predisposition to attacks. Prednisolone and colchicine both have anti-inflammatory properties, beneficial in the treatment of acute attacks.

Answer to Question 255

C

Previous pelvic surgery reduces the likelihood of successful peritoneal dialysis, adhesions often making catheter placement difficult and reducing the peritoneal surface available for dialysis. Inguinal herniae rapidly fill with peritoneal dialysate, causing patient discomfort and inefficient dialysis. Peritoneal dialysis is a good treatment for patients with diabetes mellitus, although the glucose load in the dialysate will necessitate a change in insulin dosage, which can be administered intraperitoneally. Splinting

of the diaphragm by intraperitoneal fluid can sometimes exacerbate chronic obstructive pulmonary disease, which should be considered a relative, but not absolute, contraindication. The procedure of peritoneal dialysis requires a degree of manual dexterity and would not be easy for a patient with arthritis mutilans, although various aids and adaptations can be employed.

Answer to Question 256

D

The case would be typical of post transplant lymphoproliferative disorder (PTLD), the likelihood of which is associated with the degree of previous immunosuppression. This man was exposed to potent anti-rejection therapy in the form of anti-thymocyte globulin (ATG) in addition to his baseline immunosuppressive drugs. PTLD is often driven by Epstein–Barr virus and can be treated by graded reduction in immunosuppression. It would be unusual for CMV disease to present at this time: it usually occurs much earlier in the post transplant period. Chronic rejection does not cause systemic symptoms and signs such as those described here.

Answer to Question 257

E

The history is typical of CMV infection. A transplant recipient who is at high risk of acquiring CMV disease, i.e. a CMV negative recipient of a kidney from a CMV positive donor, would routinely be given antiviral prophylaxis. Aciclovir was used in this case, which may not be the most effective agent: some units use either oral ganciclovir or valganciclovir.

Answer to Question 258

D

Lithium toxicity is common. It is rarely detected early enough for reversibility. The typical renal lesion is chronic interstitial nephritis, with a secondary focal glomerulosclerotic lesion due to hyperfiltration of remnant nephrons seen in 30% of cases.

Answer to Question 259

C

The combination of chronic analgesic use, haematuria and irregularly-shaped shrunken kidneys all suggest analgesic nephropathy. This is a specific form of chronic interstitial nephritis, more common in women and usually related to in excess of 5 years of mixed analgesic use.

Urothelial malignancy occurs in around 10% of cases and all should be investigated for this, as should anyone over 40 years of age with isolated haematuria.

Answer to Question 260
B

Ureteric reflux does not persist beyond childhood in most patients with reflux nephropathy, hence a micturating cystogram is not likely to be helpful and this test is rarely (if ever) performed in adult nephrological practice. Ultrasound is a good method of detecting the renal scars that are expected in reflux nephropathy, although it is less sensitive than intravenous urography or DMSA scanning in detecting small scars in patients with normal renal function. However, intravenous urography (or CT scanning with contrast) would not produce good quality images in this case where the degree of renal impairment would prevent adequate concentration of contrast agent for imaging.

Answer to Question 261
E

It is probably correct to say that any drug can cause an interstitial nephritis, but some do so much more commonly than others. The most likely culprits are non-steroidal anti-inflammatory agents, penicillins, proton pump inhibitors, thiazide diuretics and allopurinol, but treat all drugs – especially any started within the last six weeks – with suspicion.

Rheumatology and Clinical Immunology

Answer to Question 262
A

Pattern 1 is that of a patient with perennial rhinitis, which is commonly due to house dust mite allergy; pattern 2 is normal; pattern 3 would be typical of a patient taking antihistamines; pattern 4 of someone with dermatographism; pattern 5 is of a patient with hayfever due to grass pollen allergy.

Oral histamines should be discontinued for 4 days (4 weeks in the case of astemizole) before skin prick testing because, as shown, they can mask reactions. Areas of induration more than 3 mm in diameter greater than that of the negative control are considered to be positive: the area of erythema is not measured.

Answer to Question 263
C

The CT shows a large multilocular liver abscess. This, together with the family history and the perianal abscess, suggest an inherited neutrophil killing defect, such as chronic granulomatous disease.

The nitroblue tetrazolium (NBT) test is used as a screening test for neutrophil killing defects, when the neutrophils fail to reduce NBT that they have phagocytosed, which remains in the neutrophils as dark blue crystals.

Answer to Question 264
E

The CT scan shows soft tissue masses occupying the left nasal cavity, left ethmoid sinus, left maxillary antrum, and both orbits. The staining of neutrophils shows granular fluorescence of the cytoplasm typical of c-ANCA that in this clinical context virtually clinches the diagnosis of Wegener's granulomatosis, which would be confirmed by a specific test for antibodies directed against proteinase-3 (PR3-ANCA).

Answer to Question 265
E

Fluid A would be typical of osteoarthritis; fluid B of gout; fluid C of a non-crystal associated inflammatory arthritis (e.g. rheumatoid, reactive, psoriatic); fluid D of septic arthritis. The crystals in the joint in pseudogout are made of calcium pyrophosphate, which are rhomboid or rectangular and not needle shaped.

Answer to Question 266
D, I

The primary concern in the assessment of the acute hot joint is to exclude septic arthritis, hence diagnostic aspiration of synovial fluid is the essential urgent investigation. Grossly purulent fluid suggests sepsis; blood-stained fluid may indicate haemarthrosis but can also occur in pseudogout, which is the likeliest cause of this presentation.

An acute hot joint in an elderly person is most often due to crystal arthritis, whereas a reactive arthritis is more probable in a sexually active young adult.

Answer to Question 267
A

The history is typical of a patient with mechanical back pain, best treated by encouraging mobilisation, simple analgaesia, a graded rehabilitative exercise programme and treatment of depression (if present).

'Red flag' symptoms, requiring urgent investigation to exclude sinister pathology, include: age >55 or <18 yr, progressive pain, night pain, systemic symptoms, progressive neurological deficit, past history of malignancy or immunosuppression, and recent trauma.

Answer to Question 268
A, I

Antibody deficient patients need prompt treatment of presumed bacterial infection. Treatment should be continued for longer than normal: 14 days for an uncomplicated chest infection would be appropriate. Most infections are caused by common organisms such as haemophilus or pneumococcus: psuedomonas is unusual and mycobacterial disease rare in common variable immunodeficiency. Cultures are invaluable if there is a poor response to treatment and for guiding future antibiotic choices. For infections causing fever, routine antibody replacement should be deferred for 24–48 hours until there is a clear response to treatment, as adverse reactions are much more common in the presence of fever.

Answer to Question 269
E, I

The most likely diagnosis is avascular necrosis, the risk factors for this being corticosteroids and SLE itself, particularly in patients with anti-cardiolipin antibodies. Sepsis is less likely but possible: it must be excluded. The risk of sepsis is increased by immunosuppression, which may also modify the presentation – less fever, more insidious onset, and bloods may be normal.

This patient is at increased risk of osteoporosis but a hip fracture would be a very rare event at this age, and would usually be associated with sudden onset of pain rather than insidious onset. Osteoarthritis due to synovitis is almost never seen in SLE which produces a non-erosive arthritis.

Answer to Question 270
C

Poorly controlled asthma is an important risk factor for fatal anaphylaxis in this situation and all efforts necessary should be made to ensure that asthma is well controlled. Parents and children (when old enough) should be taught how to recognise the early symptoms and signs of anaphylaxis, how to administer self-injectable adrenaline, and should always have this available.

Answer to Question 271
D

The symptoms, signs and low C4 are suggestive of cryoglobulinaemia. Sludging of proteins at reduced temperatures – as might occur in the hands on a cold day – can cause ischaemia and sometimes vasculitis. Cryoglobulinaemia is commonly associated with hepatitis C or connective tissue disease, such as Sjögren's syndrome. The positive ANA and high globulins suggest Sjögren's in this case, but could also be associated with chronic infection, such as hepatitis C.

Since they precipitate at low temperatures, cryoglobulins should always be transported to the lab at 37°C. Failure to do this will result in a false negative result as the cryos will precipitate and be removed with the clot.

Answer to Question 272
C

Hypogammaglobulinaemia is associated with recurrent bacterial infections, most commonly of the respiratory tract. Delay of several years prior to diagnosis is usual, with associated morbidity. Patients with low immunoglobulin levels and recurrent infections should be treated with immunoglobulin replacement. More minor antibody defects, such as IgG subclass or specific antibody (to pneumococcus) defects can often be treated with appropriate vaccinations and/or prophylactic antibiotics.

Answer to Question 273
C

Hereditary angioneurotic oedema is an autosomal dominant condition caused by a deficiency of C1 esterase inhibitor, resulting in intermittent episodes of spontaneous complement activation. Clinically the patient suffers oedema of the skin and mucosal surfaces. Fatalities may occur if the airway is compromised. C4 levels are typically low during an attack but may be normal in between attacks.

Acquired angioedema is associated with allergic reactions, often associated with urticaria, and very commonly (94% of cases) drug-induced, most frequently by angiotensin-converting enzyme (ACE) inhibitors. Insect stings and foods are other predisposing factors.

Answer to Question 274
C

Acute gout is intensely inflammatory and causes severe pain, redness, swelling and disability. At least 80% of initial attacks involve a single joint, typically in the leg or foot, most often the base of the great toe (first metatarsophalangeal joint, known as podagra) or the knee. Trauma, surgery, starvation, alcohol, dietary overindulgence and ingestion of drugs, most commonly diuretics (also cyclosporin and low dose aspirin), may all promote gouty attacks. Diabetes mellitus, obesity, hyperparathyroidism and hypothyroidism are associated with gout, but rheumatoid arthritis is not associated with hyperuricaemia or gout.

Answer to Question 275

B

A history of penicillin allergy is relatively common. In most cases it is not due to a type I hypersensitivity reaction. Diagnosis of penicillin allergy crucially requires a detailed history of the drug reaction and can be confirmed by a positive skin prick test to the major and minor determinants of penicillin. Skin prick testing is carried out if there is a clinical need for penicillin treatment, e.g. treatment of infective endocarditis. A patient is unlikely to develop anaphylaxis with a negative penicillin skin prick test. The detection of penicillin specific IgE in the serum is unreliable.

Answer to Question 276

D

Although 5% of the general population have Raynaud's phenomenon, only a minority go on to develop systemic connective tissue disease. A positive ANA is the single best predictor of existing or future progression to connective tissue disease in this situation.

Answer to Question 277

A

Almost all patients with SLE have a positive ANA, which is a sensitive for SLE, but not specific. A negative result argues strongly against a diagnosis of active SLE, but does not exclude the possibility of other autoimmune diseases.

Antibodies to Sm antigen are highly specific for a diagnosis of SLE (>99%), but only about 25% of patients with SLE have anti-Sm antibodies. Anti-DNA antibodies are diagnostic of SLE (specificity > 99%), but only 60% of patients with SLE will have these antibodies. Absence of anti-DNA or anti-Sm antibodies cannot exclude SLE as a diagnosis. Anti-Ro/SS-A antibodies are found in 30% of patients with SLE. Anti-histone antibodies are identified in few SLE patients, most often those with drug-induced lupus.

Answer to Question 278

E

The recent limb weakness with pyramidal signs (upgoing plantars) in the legs in a patient with RA is very suggestive of spinal cord compression, most likely in the neck since RA primarily affects the cervical spine. The anatomic abnormalities occur as a consequence of the destruction of synovial joints, ligaments and bone, with atlantoaxial subluxation most common. Patients may experience generalised weakness, difficulty walking, paresthesias of the hands, and loss of fine dexterity. Many neurological signs may be elicited, including diffuse hyperreflexia, spasticity of the legs, a spastic gait and Babinski's sign.

Answer to Question 279

D

Antibody deficiency is typically associated with respiratory tract infections. Ask about diarrhoea and bacterial skin infections which are also common. Take a careful drug history and bear in mind the possibility of lymphoproliferative disease.

HIV infection, although primarily associated with CD4 loss, also results in antibody dysfunction leading to recurrent respiratory tract infections in some patients. Ask about features of cellular immune deficiency (oral candida, herpes simplex and zoster, warts), also about risk factors.

Recurrent bacterial chest infections, whatever their cause, will eventually result in bronchiectasis, hence the importance of early diagnosis and treatment.

Terminal complement deficiencies (C5-9) are extremely rare. Patients are well but have increased susceptibility to neisserial infection.

Smoking causes ciliary paralysis, with the resultant mucociliary dysfunction a common (and reversible) cause of recurrent respiratory tract infection.

Answer to Question 280

E

Poor adherence is a common cause of treatment failure or early relapse: directly observed therapy (DOT) may improve adherence if this is the case.

TB usually responds well to conventional treatment even if the patient is co-infected with HIV. In this situation, recurrent TB is most often caused by poor adherence (early) or reinfection (late).

Underlying IFNγ receptor/IL12 deficiency is extremely rare and is associated with disseminated disease, usually with poorly pathogenic environmental mycobacteria.

Environmental mycobacteria may occasionally grow as contaminants in culture, but it is most unusual for MTB to do so.

Answer to Question 281

B

The hallmark of all forms of C1 inhibitor deficiency is a reduced C4 with normal C3, which is a consequence of uncontrolled activation of the complement classical pathway. At this age the most likely diagnosis is acquired C1 inhibitor deficiency associated with lymphoproliferative disease or more rarely autoantibodies to C1 inhibitor.

Answer to Question 282

A

The constellation of acute symptoms is typical of a systemic allergic reaction, either anaphylaxis (if IgE mediated) or an anaphylactoid reaction (if non-IgE mediated).

Both of these reactions are due to extensive mast cell degranulation leading to release of large amounts of tryptase into the circulation. Elevated tryptase levels in this clinical context are very suggestive of an anaphylactic/anaphylactoid reaction.

This woman will need to be investigated during convalescence in an allergy clinic to determine the cause of her reaction.

Answer to Question 283

B

The most likely diagnosis in this patient is chronic idiopathic angioedema. However, the rarer C1-inhibitor deficiency has to be considered and would be excluded by a normal C4 level. The lack of any temporal relationship of his symptoms to the ingestion of any food excludes an allergic cause, which only rarely presents as chronic angioedema.

Index